A WHOLE SCHOOL APPROACH TO MENTAL HEALTH AND WELL-BEING

2ND EDITION

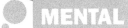

POSITIVE

MENTAL

HEALTH

POSITIVE MENTAL HEALTH

This series of texts presents a modern and comprehensive set of evidence-based strategies for promoting positive mental health in schools. There is a growing prevalence of mental ill health among children and young people within a context of funding cuts, strained services and a lack of formal training for teachers, as well as the added issues around trauma and anxiety that have developed post-Covid. The series recognises the complexity of the issues involved, the vital role that teachers play, and the current education and health policy frameworks, in order to provide practical guidance backed up by the latest research.

ACKNOWLEDGMENTS

Emma Kavanagh

Susan Woodshore

Lizzy Thornton-Dean

Helen Parry

Lauren Howard, Stour Valley Community School

School Mental Health Award Leads

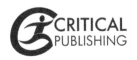

A WHOLE SCHOOL APPROACH TO MENTAL HEALTH AND WELL-BEING

2ND EDITION

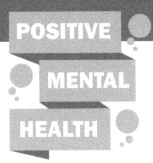

POSITIVE MENTAL HEALTH

Jonathan Glazzard and Rachel Bostwick

First published in 2018 by Critical Publishing Ltd
This second edition published in 2024

British Library Cataloguing in Publication Data
A CIP record for this book is available from the British Library

ISBN: 978-1-915713-15-5

This book is also available in the following e-book formats:

EPUB ISBN: 978-1-915713-16-2
Adobe e-book ISBN: 978-1-915713-17-9

Cover and text design by Out of House Limited
Project Management by Out of House Publishing Solutions

Critical Publishing
3 Connaught Road
St Albans
AL3 5RX

www.criticalpublishing.com

+ CONTENTS

+MEET THE SERIES EDITOR AND AUTHORS

JONATHAN GLAZZARD

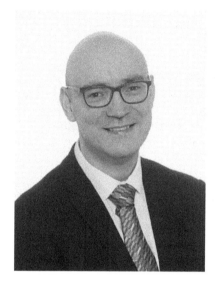

RACHEL BOSTWICK

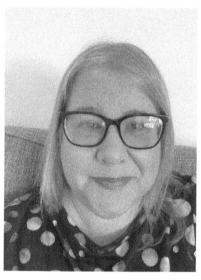

Jonathan Glazzard is the series editor for Positive Mental Health. He is the Rosalind Hollis Professor of Education for Social Justice in the School of Education at the University of Hull. Jonathan is a co-convenor of the British Educational Research Association Special Interest Group, Mental Health and Wellbeing in Education.

Rachel Bostwick is Senior Partnership and Enterprise Consultant and leads the Carnegie Centre of Excellence for Mental Health in Schools and the School Mental Health Award at Leeds Beckett University. The Award exists to strengthen the mental health of the next generation by supporting schools to make a positive change at all levels.

✛ INTRODUCTION

This book supports teachers and school leaders to develop a whole school approach to mental health. Mental health is not the same thing as mental illness. Everyone has mental health and there is a need to de-stigmatise the term. It is important for teachers and school leaders to create a school culture which enables everyone who is part of the school community to talk openly about mental health.

As a teacher or school leader you are responsible for, or will contribute to, creating a school culture which promotes positive mental health. Creating a sense of belonging for all members of the school community is important. This will help to promote well-being. Developing a curriculum which explicitly teaches children about mental health is vital for developing students' mental health literacy. Creating systems for identifying mental health needs will ensure that students do not slip through the net.

In 2021, one in six children and young people had a probable mental health need (Young Minds, 2024), representing an increase from one in ten in 2017 (DfE, DoH, 2017). These statistics demonstrate the adverse impacts of the Covid-19 global pandemic on young people's mental health. Young people are exposed to multiple risk factors which can have detrimental impacts on their mental health, and some children are more vulnerable than others. The pressures on young people appear to be increasing. They are subjected to a challenging academic curriculum and high-stakes testing, which starts in primary schools. The links between social media and mental health are also now well documented. The links between poverty and mental health are also well established. However, the causes will vary across individuals and the solutions need to be personalised to individuals rather than generic.

Following the publication of government mental health strategy in the 2017, through the publication of the document Transforming Children and Young People's Mental Health Provision: a Green Paper (DfE, DoH, 2017), many schools have implemented actions to improve the mental health provision that is available. These actions include developing the role of Designated Senior Lead for Mental Health, implementing a whole school approach to support well-being and mental health, investing in staff training and developing a mental health curriculum. The government has invested in Mental Health Support Teams through introducing training programmes for the role of the Education Mental Health Practitioner (EMHP). However, more still needs to be done. Currently, waiting lists to access specialist services are too long and too many young people do not meet the threshold criteria for referral. Consequently, support often comes too late or not at all. The responsibility is often placed on schools to address pupils' mental health needs, yet teachers feel inadequately prepared to undertake this task.

This book supports you to develop your mental health provision. However, new challenges will continue to emerge to which schools will need to respond. This illustrates the need for teachers to continually update their knowledge and the need for high-quality professional development to enable them to do this.

It is important to avoid stereotypes. Children and young people who are born into areas of social deprivation will not inevitably develop a mental health need. Children from high-income families do develop mental health needs. While some groups of young people are more vulnerable than others, not all care experienced children and young people or those living in care will have mental health needs. Children who are polite, high performing, well behaved and dressed smartly may have mental health needs but these may be invisible. Young people may appear to be coping well but may be hiding serious mental health needs. Systems of identification in schools need to catch all these children.

This book provides a concise text for busy teachers and school leaders detailing what you need to know to help inform your school's approach to mental health. It contains a number of features that highlight particular types of information. Research boxes are indicated by a magnifying glass symbol. There are also professional links, case studies and critical questions along with helpful objectives, checklists and summaries.

Jonathan Glazzard and Rachel Bostwick

+ CHAPTER 1

WHAT IS MENTAL HEALTH?

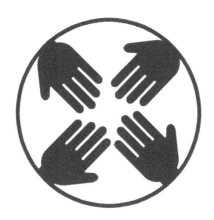

CHAPTER OBJECTIVES

By the end of this chapter you will understand:

+ what mental health is;
+ your legal responsibilities in relation to supporting children and young people with mental health needs;
+ types of mental health needs;
+ the role of schools in promoting positive mental health in children and young people.

INTRODUCTION

This chapter outlines what we mean by mental health and provides an overview of the contribution that primary and secondary schools can make to the promotion of good mental health. Evidence suggests that mental health needs appear to be increasing (NHS Digital, 2023). One in six children has a probable mental health condition (Young Minds, 2023), and girls are particularly at risk of developing a low sense of well-being (Danby and Hamilton, 2016). While this is concerning, it is also possible that increased public awareness of mental health has resulted in more effective identification and diagnosis processes (Burton, 2014).

Research demonstrates that there are multiple risk factors which result in mental health needs. These include: income inequality; relationship breakdown; parental conflict; parental health; school expectations; bullying, including digital bullying and concerns about body image (Bor et al, 2014; Danby and Hamilton, 2016). Other risk factors include low self-esteem, abuse, neglect, socio-economic disadvantage, peer influences and grief or loss (DfE, 2016).

Research demonstrates that an increasing number of children and young people are demonstrating self-harm, phobia, depression, anxiety, substance misuse, attachment disorders, conduct disorders and eating disorders (DfE, 2014; Dickins, 2014; Sisask et al, 2014). There is evidence to suggest that children and young people with special educational needs are more at risk of developing mental health conditions (Lindsay and Dockrell, 2012) and those exposed to multiple risk factors demonstrate a significantly increased risk (Weare, 2010).

Children and young people with mental health needs are at risk of being absent from school and underachieving academically (DH, 2014). The 2023 Ofsted report highlights the issue of the increasing number of children and young people who are presenting with emotionally based school avoidance and the increasing use of part-time timetables for pupils who are presenting with anxiety (Ofsted, 2023). While schools can have a positive impact by developing universal approaches for all pupils and addressing the specific needs of those who require targeted support, it is important to emphasise that schools cannot meet the mental health needs of all pupils in isolation (O'Hara, 2014). Some pupils will require specialist provision, particularly in cases where needs are complex and where there is risk of harm to the child. Ofsted has highlighted the detrimental impact that shortages of specialist mental health services is having on children, young people and schools (Ofsted, 2023).

WHAT IS MENTAL HEALTH?

The following perspective has been adopted by the World Health Organisation:

Mental health is a state of mental well-being that enables people to cope with the stresses of life, realise their abilities, learn well and work well, and contribute to their community ... Mental health is more than the absence of mental disorders. It exists on a complex continuum, which is experienced differently from one person to the next, with varying degrees of difficulty and distress and potentially very different social and clinical outcomes.

(WHO, 2022)

Contemporary perspectives on health position mental health as a positive concept rather than as a deficit attribute within a person (Weare, 2010; Weare and Markham, 2005). Thus, mental health has been conceptualised as a continuum, with good mental health at one end of the spectrum and mental illness at the other end (Danby and Hamilton, 2016). It is critical that children and young people understand that everyone has mental health and that this lies somewhere along this continuum; there will be times when most people need more support than at other times (Prever, 2006) and being able to recognise this is crucial in order to make positive changes. Thus, helping young people to understand firstly, that mental health exists within a state of flux and secondly, that they can largely control it, can provide them with a sense of agency. Mental health moves along a continuum and is influenced by a range of social, biological and psychological factors. Helping children to understand what factors they can change and what individual and external resources they can draw on for support are important ways of empowering young people to take greater responsibility for their own mental health.

The physical, social, psychological and emotional aspects of health overlap and interrelate (Danby and Hamilton, 2016). Children and young people's mental health is influenced by the quality of relationships they form with peers and adults (Thapa et al, 2013). This is known as social connectedness (Aldridge and Chesney, 2018). Engagement in physical activity can also improve mental health. However, while social connections and physical activity can improve mental health, having good mental health can also impact on the extent to which young people choose to participate in establishing social connections and physical activity.

Tabloid coverage can result in negative assumptions and stigma (Barber, 2012) in relation to mental health. This can lead to practitioners and parents forming a deficit view which associates mental health with mental illness (Holstrom, 2013; Time to Change, 2015). Schools play an important role in reducing stigma by helping children to understand that mental health is a fundamental aspect of overall health. By mainstreaming conversations about mental health, schools can help young people to understand that mental health is not something to be ashamed of. The stigmatisation of mental health can have detrimental effects (Danby and Hamilton, 2016) because it can reduce the willingness of individuals to talk about their needs.

School leaders and teachers have a responsibility for providing safe, caring and nurturing environments so that all pupils can thrive. However, it has been argued that there is a danger of viewing young children as psychologically and emotionally vulnerable (Ecclestone, 2014, 2015), particularly when they display specific reactions to daily experiences which influence their emotions. Schools therefore play an important role in promoting young people's resilience to adverse situations so that they can 'bounce back' from these.

Certain risk factors are linked to mental health needs. These include:

+ *parental conflict;*

+ *income inequality;*

+ *parental relationship breakdown;*

+ *parental health;*

+ *cyberbullying;*

+ *school expectations;*

+ *special educational needs/additional learning needs;*

+ *school environment.*

(Danby and Hamilton, 2016, p 91)

CRITICAL QUESTIONS

+ Some life experiences are more challenging than others and will demand greater resilience to respond to them. What experiences might these include?

+ What contributions can role models make to reducing stigma about mental health?

+ What factors can protect against young people developing mental health needs?

BIOPSYCHOSOCIAL MODEL OF HEALTH

The biopsychosocial mode of health (Engel, 1977) demonstrates that our overall health is affected by a combination of biological, social and psychological factors. These factors often interact. For example, social factors (such as isolation) can impact on psychological factors (for example, our emotional well-being or anxiety), and poor emotional well-being could result in increased blood pressure (biological factors). The model is shown in Figure 1.1.

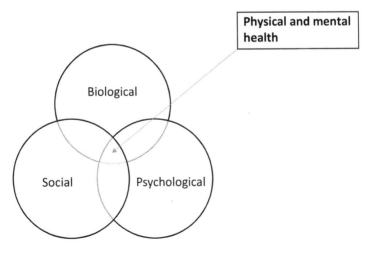

Figure 1.1. The biopsychosocial model of health (adapted from Engel, 1977)

The model demonstrates that physical and mental health can be caused by a range of overlapping factors.

MENTAL HEALTH DIAGRAM

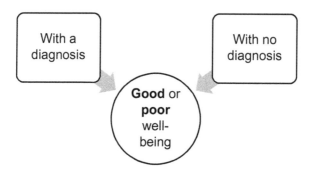

Figure 1.2. Well-being diagram (adapted from Mental Health First Aid England (MHFA), (2018)

Individuals may obtain a diagnosis of poor mental health. However, many individuals may have poor mental health but do not have a diagnosis. Diagnoses can be self-diagnosed or medically diagnosed. Self-diagnosis is also used when individuals describe their mental health as good or poor.

CRITICAL QUESTIONS

+ What factors might influence a person's decision to seek a diagnosis of mental ill-health?
+ Why might some individuals be reluctant to seek a diagnosis?

THE STRESS CONTAINER

Stress is not a mental health condition, but the experience of stress can result in anxiety and other mental health conditions. It is unrealistic to aim to live a life free of stress. Some stress in our lives can also help us to achieve our goals, stay motivated and be productive. We all have a 'stress container' (MHFA, 2018) which is our capacity for coping with stress. This is shown in Figure 1.3.

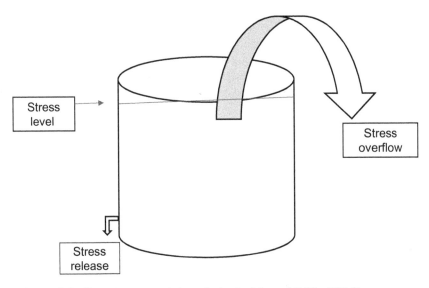

Figure 1.3. The stress container (adapted from MHFA, 2018)

Our stress container can only hold a certain amount of stress before it overloads. The capacity of the container will vary across individuals. If the container is full, we need to release some of the stress before we start to demonstrate our 'stress signature'. We all have a unique stress signature. The stress signature is the unique emotional, behavioural and social changes that we demonstrate as a reaction to extreme stress.

CRITICAL QUESTIONS

The stress container

+ How might you describe your personal stress signature?

+ What strategies might you use to release stress from your stress container?

SELF-ESTEEM AND MENTAL HEALTH

Mruk's model of self-esteem demonstrates that our overall self-esteem is made up of self-worth (our view of ourselves) and self-competence (how well we complete challenges and tasks). The model is shown in Figure 1.4.

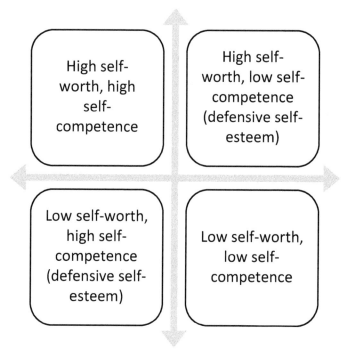

Figure 1.4. Two-dimensional model of self-esteem (adapted from Mruk, 1999)

The vertical axis represents self-worth, and the horizontal axis represents self-competence. To achieve overall high self-esteem, individuals need to have both high self-worth and high self-competence. Where there is a mismatch between self-worth and self-competence, this results in defensive self-esteem and individuals in these two quadrants can demonstrate signs of poor mental health. Individuals who are low in both dimensions (self-worth and self-competence) are also at risk of developing mental ill-health.

CRITICAL QUESTIONS

+ How might children and young people present in each of the four quadrants?

+ Where would you position yourself on the matrix? Explain your reasons.

+ Is it possible to be high in both dimensions and have poor mental health? Explain your response.

LEGAL RESPONSIBILITIES

The following legislation or guidance places a duty on schools to safeguard and promote the welfare of children and young people:

+ Section 175 of the Education Act 2002 duty applies to maintained schools.

+ The Education (Independent School Standards) Regulations 2014 applies to independent schools (which include free schools and academies).

+ The Non-Maintained Special Schools (England) Regulations 2015 place a duty on non-maintained special schools to promote the welfare of children and young people.

+ The Sexual Offences Act 2003 states that it is an offence for a person aged 18 or over (eg teacher, youth worker) to have a sexual relationship with a child under 18 where that person is in a position of trust in respect of that child, even if the relationship is consensual.

+ All schools must have regard to the following document: *Keeping Children Safe in Education: Statutory Guidance for Schools and Colleges* (DfE, 2023).

+ The Equality Act 2010: schools must prevent direct or indirect discrimination of individuals with protected characteristics. Disability is one protected characteristic, and this includes mental health conditions. This legislation places a duty on schools to provide reasonable adjustments to ensure equality of opportunity for individuals with protected characteristics. It is important to remember the multi-sectional nature of protected characteristics and thus, individuals may have one or more of these.

+ The *Special Educational Needs and Disability Code of Practice: 0 to 25 Years* (DfE/DoH, 2015): mental health is now recognised for the first time as a special educational need and schools have a duty to work in partnership with pupils, parents and external agencies to support pupils' mental health needs. The code emphasises the importance of early identification and intervention for all those with identified special educational needs and disabilities.

CRITICAL QUESTIONS

To meet these duties how might schools:

+ create a culture which promotes a sense of belonging?

+ develop approaches to support the identification of mental health needs?

+ develop the curriculum so that mental health is a taught aspect of it?

+ develop policies on teaching, learning, assessment and behaviour management which reduce the risk of mental health needs occurring?

+ develop approaches for working with parents, carers and external agencies to ensure that the needs of the child are met?

+ develop approaches to monitoring the impact of interventions?

+ develop mechanisms for providing children and young people with mental health needs with a voice so that they can participate in decision-making?

+ develop approaches to professional development in mental health for all staff?

THE IMPACT OF COVID-19 ON YOUNG PEOPLE'S MENTAL HEALTH

Evidence suggests that some children and young people's mental health and well-being has been adversely impacted as a result of the global pandemic, although the effects were experienced differently across different groups of children. Research by Young Minds (2021) found that the Covid-19 pandemic made some children and young people deeply anxious, some had started to self-harm and others were experiencing panic attacks and had lost motivation and hope for the future. The pandemic resulted in multiple pressures, especially for those who had been bereaved or experienced other trauma during this time. Since the pandemic, the prevalence of mental ill-health in children and young people has increased. Recent research by Newlove-Delgado et al (2023) found that:

+ The prevalence of a probable mental disorder in children aged 8 to 16 years rose between 2017 and 2020, from 12.5 per cent in 2017 to 17.1 per cent in 2020.

+ Children aged 8 to 16 years with a probable mental disorder were seven times more likely to be absent from school.

+ Children aged 8 to 16 years with a probable mental disorder were more than twice as likely to be experiencing poverty.

MENTAL HEALTH AND ACADEMIC ATTAINMENT

Research indicates that well-planned and well-implemented opportunities for supporting the well-being of students can positively affect academic outcomes (Greenberg et al, 2003; Gumora and Arsenio, 2002; Malecki and Elliott, 2002; Teo et al, 1996; Welsh et al, 2001; Wentzel, 1993; Wood, 2006; Zins et al, 2004). According to Sammons (2007), there are strong relationships between student behaviour, attainment and learning and their social and emotional development. Due to the relationships between mental health, academic success and life opportunities, schools have a critical role to play in promoting students' mental well-being (Clausson and Berg, 2008; Cushman et al, 2011).

CRITICAL QUESTIONS

+ Do you agree that schools have an important role to play in promoting students' well-being? Explain your answer to this.

+ Should schools prioritise students' academic development or their well-being?

MENTAL HEALTH IN PRIMARY SCHOOLS

The following section outlines the common needs which you may notice in primary schools. There are other needs mentioned later in this chapter that may occur in primary schools but more commonly occur during adolescence.

TRAUMA

According to Bessel van der Kolk (2014), *'We have learned that trauma is not just an event that took place sometime in the past; it is also the imprint left by that experience on mind, brain and body. This imprint has ongoing consequences for how the human organism manages to survive in the present'*.

Children who have experienced trauma may demonstrate the following symptoms:

+ difficulties in establishing social connections;
+ anxiety;
+ difficulties with concentration;
+ self-soothing strategies;
+ conduct disorders;
+ being quiet and withdrawn;
+ emotional and social regulation difficulties;
+ emotionally based school avoidance;
+ developmental delay.

Some schools are trauma-informed schools. Staff are specifically trained in how to implement these approaches and the approaches are used across the whole school. Trauma-informed pedagogies are sensitive, compassionate and empathetic. Children's behaviours are viewed as a form of communication rather than a sign of defiance and there is a strong emphasis on de-escalation techniques and the explicit teaching of social and emotional regulation skills. Trauma may arise from weak attachments with carers, loss and bereavement or from experiencing or witnessing abuse, war, poverty and community-related disasters such as flooding. This is not an exhaustive list.

CONDUCT DISORDERS

Children with conduct disorders may demonstrate verbal and physical aggression, defiance and anti-social behaviour. They may need support to understand what is meant by socially accepted behaviour and the impact of their behaviour on others. Approaches used in schools to support children with conduct disorders may reflect a behaviourist approach which emphasises the use of rewards and sanctions. Some children may require a highly individual rewards and sanctions system which differs from the system used for all pupils. Behaviourist approaches focus on the consequences of behaviour rather than the causes. In contrast, an alternative approach stems from a branch of psychology known as humanism. Humanism attempts to focus on developing the child's sense of self through improving their self-concept and self-esteem. It focuses on helping the child to recognise their strengths and is underpinned by the work of Maslow (1943) and Rogers (1951) who argued that a positive sense of self is essential to enable an individual to achieve their full potential.

ANXIETY

Anxiety is a group of related conditions, including phobias, General Anxiety Disorder (GAD), Post-Traumatic Stress Disorder (PTSD) and Obsessive Compulsive Disorder (OCD). Anxiety disorders range in type and severity. Anxiety may be related to a specific phobia, for example a fear of an object, or situation. Children may become anxious in unfamiliar situations and may be anxious in some situations but not in others. Some children may be anxious all the time. In addition, anxiety might result from separation from a significant other. Children with anxiety may display a range of symptoms. These include fearfulness, irritability, panic, breathlessness and sleep deprivation (DfE, 2016).

Ofsted's annual report has identified the following concerns:

+ *Some schools are struggling to manage ordinary pupil anxiety or, more rarely, not helping pupils to access support for more serious mental health needs.*

+ *Schools report increased staff anxiety because staff are not confident about responding to mental health needs without timely Child and Adolescent Mental Health (CAMHS) support.*

+ *Pupil anxiety and other mental health problems have increased.*

+ *Inspections are showing more and more pupils spending part of their week outside education and anxiety is a contributory factor.*

(Ofsted, 2023)

ATTACHMENT DISORDERS

The work of Bowlby (1969) helped to demonstrate the significance of positive attachments between children and their primary caregivers. In cases where loving, caring and secure attachments are not formed because of the family context, this can have a detrimental impact on the child's sense of self and their behaviour. Children with attachment disorders may be withdrawn, demonstrate anti-social behaviour, have low confidence and a negative perception of their abilities. Forming positive and secure relationships with children is essential, particularly in cases where attachments with their primary caregivers are weak, non-existent or absent. Some children with attachment disorders may benefit from interventions which help them to develop a positive sense of self.

CRITICAL QUESTIONS

+ What situations in school may result in a child feeling anxious?

+ What are the advantages and disadvantages of supporting conduct disorders through a behaviourist approach?

+ What are the advantages and disadvantages of supporting conduct disorders through a solution-focused approach which involves the child in setting goals and supports them in recognising their own strengths?

CASE STUDY

One primary school decided to introduce a universal approach to supporting children's well-being. Rather than focusing only on children who presented needs, they used the resources from the Head Start

16

resources with all children. They selected resources from the toolkit: www.corc.uk.net/media/1506/primary-school-measures_310317_forweb.pdf.

They decided to adopt the feelings survey and the resilience survey, which all children completed once a term. This allowed teachers to identify any children with specific needs and provide appropriate support, but it also enabled senior leaders to identify differences in feelings and resilience between specific groups of children (for example, gender, ethnicity, age and special educational needs).

Research by Danby and Hamilton (2016) found that primary practitioners tended to focus on developing children's understanding of feelings and promoting their resilience. However, they were reluctant to use the term 'mental health' with children as they perceived this to be an unsuitable term to use with children. This can result in children forming negative views about mental health, which can result in stigma. The danger is that these attitudes can make discussions about mental health awkward and it becomes taboo.

CRITICAL QUESTIONS

+ What are your views on the use of the term 'mental health' with young children?

+ What are the benefits of using the term 'mental health' with young children?

+ What issues may result from using the term 'mental health' with young children?

+ How might you overcome these issues?

MENTAL HEALTH IN SECONDARY SCHOOLS

This section addresses common mental health needs in secondary schools. Needs that have been identified earlier in this chapter may also be evident in secondary schools. Specific mental health needs may also co-exist alongside other mental health needs or may exist alongside other identified needs.

MOOD DISORDERS

Mood disorders include depression and bipolar disorder. While depression is a form of low mood, there are differences between the two. Low mood may be characterised by a feeling of sadness or disappointment, but depression is more severe. It is more persistent and it may affect normal daily functioning.

Bipolar disorder is a disorder in which the mood can become extremely high or low, with episodes lasting for several days or weeks. Characteristics include extreme mood swings and mania. Depression exists along a spectrum ranging from mild to severe. It can fluctuate depending on personal experiences and can affect a child's ability to learn. Children may become withdrawn, tearful, and demonstrate persistent low mood. They may demonstrate decreased energy, sleeplessness and loss of appetite. Engagement in physical activity, social activity and a healthy diet can alleviate depression. Supporting a young person to experience success can also help. It is important to encourage young people to talk about how they feel and for responsible adults to become good listeners. You will need to demonstrate patience and empathy.

SELF-HARM

Self-harm is a behaviour and not an illness. It can be used as a coping strategy in response to emotional pain and is often carried out secretly. It is not an attention-seeking behaviour and individuals who self-harm sometimes experience a feeling of being emotionally numb. Self-harm might therefore be a behaviour which enables individuals to feel something. Self-harm can include hitting, cutting, burning, picking skin, pulling hair, over-dosing and self-strangulation. It is particularly worrying that children can now access websites which promote self-harm and normalise it, and it is also a concern that the process of self-harm can now be viewed through live streaming on the internet. Self-harm may co-exist alongside other conditions such as stress, anxiety and depression, and it might be a response to these conditions. It may also be a response to abuse, neglect and other traumatic incidents.

The personal, social and emotional (PSE) curriculum should introduce children to self-harm and this topic should be addressed sensitively. In addition, schools will need to decide when to introduce this content in the curriculum and content should be age-appropriate.

If children and young people disclose to you that they are engaging in self-harm, it is important to listen to them and respond with empathy. They may have chosen to self-harm because they have experienced trauma and the process of self-harming may be a way of managing their emotions. Although you may be concerned about their actions, responding in a negative way by highlighting the associated risks is unlikely to be beneficial. Acknowledge what they are saying to you and demonstrate empathy and compassion. Talk with them, not at them and then review with them what will happen next. If they have asked you to keep the information confidential, this may not be possible, especially if you are concerned about risks to the child. In these circumstances, discuss with them why you need to pass the information on to others, who you will tell, what information you will share and what will happen next. Refer the information to the Designated Safeguarding Lead (DSL). If you suspect that a child is self-harming but they do not disclose it, you have a duty to refer this information to the DSL. It is important to remember that self-harm is not just something that adolescents do. Young children also self-harm but it may manifest differently.

EATING DISORDERS

Eating disorders include anorexia nervosa and bulimia nervosa. Both disorders may be associated with a desire to be thin and body image concerns. Binge eating disorder is also another eating disorder. Anorexia is an intense fear of gaining weight, accompanied by extreme efforts to control weight. Bulimia includes episodes of binge eating, commonly followed by episodes of purging. Binge eating disorder involves eating a large amount of food in a short amount of time, but is not followed by purging. Eating disorders might also arise as a response to trauma. Signs could include sudden loss of appetite, loss of weight, vomiting after food, anxiety or depression. Children with eating disorders may require specialist support from the health profession.

Children's body image may be negatively influenced by advertising and the media (including social media) and peer influences. Research indicates that advertisements often portray idealised images of beauty (Frith, 2017), which impacts negatively on body confidence. Females are often depicted through images of slender bodies which are used to represent beauty and perfection (Frith, 2017). Images and messages about 'perfect' bodies are internalised, and this can lead to children and young people making unrealistic comparisons between the media images and their own bodies. This can result in low body esteem.

While the research suggests that females may be more prone to poor body image than males, boys and young men can also be affected (British Youth Council, 2017). Advertisements which portray the perfect male body often depict muscular strength as a characteristic of the ideal male body. Research suggests that this can result in males developing an obsession with muscle building, as a result of developing body dissatisfaction (British Youth Council, 2017).

Schools need to address the theme of body image through the PSE curriculum. Children should be supported to challenge the stereotypes that they are exposed to in the media. Additionally, the science curriculum will introduce children to the importance of a healthy balanced diet. The processes outlined above for referring concerns should be followed. If the child discloses that they have an eating disorder, it is important to demonstrate empathy, compassion and to listen to them. The discussion should be non-judgemental.

SUBSTANCE ABUSE

Substance abuse can include alcohol, drugs and prescribed medications. Substance abuse increases the risk of developing a mental health condition because some substances can also act as depressants, for example, alcohol. Substance abuse also increases impulsivity and can also result in distortions to thinking. People who are abusing substances might start to catastrophise or focus on negative details. They may interpret things in a negative way or they might start to blame themselves for things.

SUICIDE

The extent of death by suicide in the UK is a concern. Significantly more males than females die by suicide and LGBTQ+ individuals are more likely to attempt suicide than those who are not LGBTQ+ (MHFA, 2018).

In addition:

+ *Suicide is one of the leading causes of death in children and young people.*

+ *Suicide may be linked to many factors, including poor mental health and adverse childhood experiences.*

+ Suicide represents the extreme endpoint of mental ill-health in children and young people. Many more young people either have suicidal ideation, attempt suicide, and a greater number still self-harm.

(Royal College of Paediatrics and Child Health, 2020, https://stateofchildhealth. rcpch.ac.uk/evidence/mental-health/suicide/)

CRITICAL QUESTIONS

+ What contribution might the examination system in secondary schools make to students' mental health needs?

+ Why might adolescence be a particularly vulnerable time for young people?

+ How might peer pressure influence mental health during adolescence?

+ How might social media influence mental health during adolescence?

+ Why do you think more males than females die by suicide?

+ Why is the LGBTQ+ population particularly at risk of dying by suicide?

+ How might you structure a conversation with a child or young person who discloses to you that they are thinking of dying by suicide and what actions would you take next?

CASE STUDY

A secondary school decided to use the Warwick-Edinburgh Mental Well-being Scale, the perceived stress scale and the student resilience survey from the Head Start resources: www.corc.uk.net/media/1506/primary-school-measures_310317_forweb.pdf.

The stress scale was used with all students in Years 10 and 11 while they were undertaking their GCSE courses. The students completed it once a term. The other two surveys were completed by all students at the start of each academic year. The perceived stress scale was particularly useful as it allowed teachers to identify students who felt they were experiencing stress. The pastoral leader then met with these students to discuss the factors that had contributed to them feeling stressed. Strategies were established by the school to support these students at a critical time in their academic development. Students were asked to make suggestions of strategies which they felt would help them, and the pastoral leader also suggested strategies for alleviating stress. One of the outcomes was the introduction of a dedicated room for students to use for revision purposes in preparation for the examinations. This was particularly useful for students who did not have adequate revision space at home. Some students were given planners to help them organise their workload, and all students who perceived they were experiencing stress were provided with lessons on stress management. This included mindfulness activities and physical activity sessions during the school day.

Research indicates that an engaging environment that supports the active participation of young people in the school plays a protective role in relation to physical, social and emotional health, and enables young people to thrive academically (Butcher, 2010; Noble and Toft, 2010). Central to such thinking is the concept of school 'connectedness'. This is where students believe that adults in the school care about them as individuals and care about their learning (Blum and Libbey, 2004). Greater school connectedness reduces the likelihood that young people will engage in health-compromising behaviours and increases the likelihood of academic success (Klem and Connell, 2004). Research has also shown that young people who report high levels of school connectedness report lower levels of emotional distress and risk-taking behaviours (Blum and Libbey, 2004). Research has shown that students who lack social and emotional skills often become less connected to school as they get older. This lack of connection has been found to have a negative impact on their academic attainment, behaviour and health (Durlak et al, 2011). Students with low school connectedness are two to three times more likely to experience mental health symptoms compared to more connected peers (Glover et al, 1998).

SUMMARY

Teachers are not mental health experts. However, there is much that schools can do to promote positive mental health. Fundamental to this is the role of school culture in establishing a climate where students feel that they belong. The role of teachers and other practitioners in establishing positive relationships with students is critical to establishing school connectedness. It appears that the prevalence of mental health needs among children and young people is increasing. However, mental health should no longer be seen as a stigma; it is something that everyone has, and it is not synonymous with mental illness. Young people are subjected to the influences of the societies in which they live. Their mental health is influenced by a range of complex social, environmental, cultural and political factors which are not always positive. There are no quick fixes, but we can start by supporting young people to understand what mental health is and we can provide them with some tools to help them develop positive well-being. Schools play a vital role in relation to both identification of needs and intervention. Mental health and academic achievement are inter-related and the most effective schools place student well-being at the heart of any school improvement plan.

CHECKLIST

This chapter has addressed:

✓ what is meant by mental health;

✓ the role of schools in promoting a positive culture;

✓ key mental health needs;

✓ ways in which schools might assess young people's well-being.

FURTHER READING

Adelman, H S and Taylor, L (2015) *Mental Health in Schools: Engaging Learners, Preventing Problems, and Improving Schools.* New York: Skyhorse Publishing.

Holt, M K and Grills, A E (2015) *Critical Issues in School-based Mental Health: Evidence-based Research, Practice, and Interventions.* New York: Routledge.

✚ CHAPTER 2

PROMOTING A WHOLE SCHOOL APPROACH TO WELL-BEING AND MENTAL HEALTH

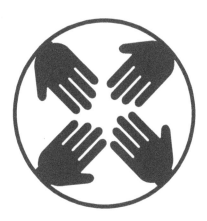

CHAPTER OBJECTIVES

After reading this chapter you will understand:

+ what a whole school approach to mental health looks like;

+ the importance of school culture and leadership;

+ the importance of taking care of staff mental health;

+ how to implement a whole school approach to mental health.

INTRODUCTION

Teachers are not health professionals. The key role of a teacher is to educate children and young people. They are not trained to diagnose mental health conditions or to deliver psychological interventions. However, they spend much more time working with young people than professionals from health or social care services. Therefore, they are well placed to *identify* possible mental health needs but they are not qualified to diagnose a mental health condition.

The whole school approach was developed by Public Health England (2021). It is designed to be preventative. If implemented well, it should reduce the number of children and young people who need to be referred to specialist mental health services. Some mental health issues are temporary or triggered by certain factors, and many people experience stress and anxiety. Others have greater permanency. Reducing the triggers will help to alleviate problems. In cases where problems are more persistent, teachers should be alert to the signs, which may indicate the need for referral and/or targeted interventions.

This chapter addresses ways in which schools can promote a whole school approach to mental health. We consider the role of the school culture, the policies of the school and the curriculum in facilitating positive mental health for children, young people and adults who work in schools.

THE WHOLE SCHOOL APPROACH

Implementing a whole school approach demonstrates a strategic commitment to mental health and well-being. The model is divided into eight strands as shown in Figure 2.1.

The Whole School Approach is intended to be a preventative model. If schools and colleges implement the model, this should reduce the prevalence of mental ill-health and lead to a reduction in the number of children and young people who need to be referred to specialist mental health services. The role of the school/college leadership team in championing mental health and well-being is central to the model.

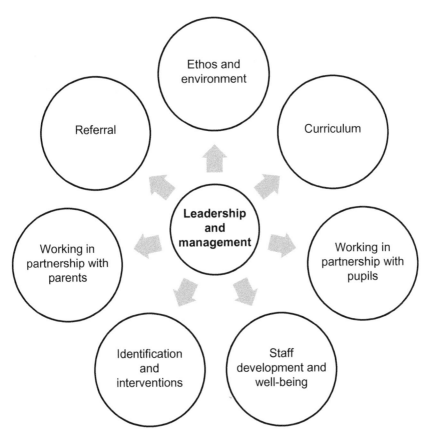

Figure 2.1. The whole school approach to mental health (adapted from Public Health England, 2021)

LEADERSHIP AND MANAGEMENT

Leadership teams in schools are the driving forces for school improvement. This strand of the whole school approach requires school leaders to champion mental health and well-being. Leaders should develop policies for staff and pupil well-being which outline how the whole school approach will be implemented. Appointing a Designated Senior Lead (DSL) for mental health demonstrates a strategic commitment to this strand of work. In addition, nominating a school governor to work with the DSL will ensure that the mental health provision in the school can be robustly monitored. To support the implementation of the whole school approach, school leaders need to ensure that there is a robust system for identifying mental health needs in the school. In addition, leaders need to invest in providing staff training so that staff can identify the signs and symptoms of mental ill-health and feel confident in talking to pupils about mental health. Leaders need to ensure that there is a curriculum in place which introduces pupils to mental health content. They are also responsible for ensuring that pupils' mental health needs are met through a range of interventions and for safeguarding children.

CASE STUDY

ARTHUR MELLOWS VILLAGE COLLEGE, PETERBOROUGH

Following the Covid-19 pandemic and during the academic year of 2021–2022, mental health and well-being became a core focus within our large, 11–18 College. With 250 staff and 1700 students, we wanted to develop strategies to support the day-to-day well-being of all and also to explore the culture of our setting to ensure that mental health and well-being was a priority. We had identified a number of risk factors affecting staff and students, which included increased sickness absence, anxiety and stress, all of which was impacting on overall satisfaction and happiness within the College.

We have since recruited a Senior Leader whose core responsibilities include mental health and well-being and they will first evaluate practice and then create a strategy plan. This has involved signing up to the Well-being Charter and then subsequently bidding for DfE funding to complete the Senior Mental Health Lead training with Carnegie Centre of Excellence for Mental Health in Schools. This training was extremely useful for building a strategy plan, as well as gaining insight from other colleagues at well-being conferences and in the online forums.

The Designated Mental Health Lead created an action plan that focused on curriculum, culture, surveys, student feedback, parental engagement and staff support as well as reviewing and/or writing policies which clearly outlined our intent. This plan was then actioned over the course of three years and is now fully embedded within the school culture. It has since been extended and the work around this is now used across our Multi-Academy Trust. In July 2023, we were awarded the Silver Award for Mental Health from Carnegie Centre of Excellence and have been invited to speak at the National Schools and Academies Show by Minds Ahead as well as PIXL.

The impact of having a whole school approach to mental health and well-being has been crucial for the development of our College and provision for students. It is embedded within everyday life, whether through social media, curriculum, examinations, performance management, charity events or engagement with parents. All of our staff and students are part of the work we do and we all feel immensely proud of how we support each other and make the College a supportive place to be.

CASE STUDY

QUEEN ERSKINE STEWART MELVILLE SCHOOLS

What is the priority?

The priority is to improve communication and strategy as, with over 2500 pupils across two sites and three provisions, this can be a challenge.

How did the school address this?

In 2021, our Principal launched a new Well-being Policy Committee, now chaired by our Director of People. We spent the first year as an open committee conducting an audit and sharing ideas, and have now largely decentralised into functional workstreams. These workstreams include guidance structure, partnerships, training and education, voice, well-being environments, and a centre for excellence and research.

Staff have visited schools across Britain to explore good practice. This led to school areas trialling new initiatives, such as morning check-ins and Smart School Council in our Junior School, and improving pupil voice. We also now use both internal and external surveys to track, monitor and, crucially, act on pupils' well-being data. This formalisation of procedures has helped us to undertake more early interventions with pupils. We have converted more spaces into calming areas and have pioneered new VR technology for transitions, with marked impact. Inspired to encourage others to increase the profile of well-being, we are now hosting a conference for educators from across Scotland.

What was the impact?

There is still more to do, but this Committee has become a sounding board for new ideas and has started to make a difference to students.

It has helped us have a sense of common goals, a clearer idea of where we want to be, and the impetus to get there.

ETHOS AND ENVIRONMENT

Research demonstrates that the physical, social and emotional environment in the school impacts on young people's physical, emotional and mental health and well-being as well as impacting on academic attainment (Jamal et al, 2013). The school ethos relates to the 'feel' of a school and central to this is the way in which members of the school community are treated. Critical to the development of a positive school ethos is the school vision. The vision should be underpinned by a set of values which demonstrate the school's commitment to challenging all forms of discrimination. The school's commitment to promoting democracy, respect and equality of opportunity for all members of the school community should be a key aspect of the vision and values. Through the vision and values, schools can also demonstrate a commitment to fostering a sense of belonging for everyone in the school community. Differences between individuals should be viewed as positive and there should be a climate of mutual trust and respect. School cultures which promote divisions between people, fear and secrecy are not positive places in which to work and learn.

In ensuring a positive school ethos, leaders need to ensure that children and young people are kept safe from discrimination, harassment and bullying. All schools are required to have robust policies and approaches for addressing bullying and inspectors evaluate these as part of school inspections. A culture of safeguarding ensures that pupils can enjoy coming to school and that they can be confident that adults will keep them safe and protect them from harm. Establishing a culture of safeguarding will reduce the prevalence of mental ill-health and enable pupils to thrive.

In establishing a positive ethos, leaders must also promote a culture of respect. One way of addressing this is to increase the visibility of different identities within the curriculum and within the school environment. Exposing pupils to diverse children's literature is one way of ensuring that race, ethnicity, gender, sexual orientation and disability are characteristics that are positively affirmed. Pupils should be exposed to a diverse range of characters, authors and poets in the literature that they read. Pupils should be introduced to the achievements of significant individuals, past and present, from minority or global majority groups within the subject curriculum and the subject curriculum should also introduce pupils to important topics, including Windrush, LGBT+ history, disability history and the changing role of women in British society. Increasing the visibility of diverse identities ensures that pupils' diverse identities are represented in the school curriculum, in books and through displays. Displays around the school can include positive messaging about mental health and can also be used to signpost pupils so that they know how to access support. A range of children's literature exists which explicitly addresses mental health through stories. These stories can be used to introduce pupils to conversations about mental health.

Leaders also need to create a positive ethos for staff. Staff thrive when they feel trusted, are valued, experience a sense of belonging and when they work within collaborative cultures. Leaders should ensure that staff are protected from bullying and harassment and introduce approaches to reduce unnecessary workload. Fundamentally, staff who work in schools are adults and they should be treated as such. Hierarchical approaches to leadership and cultures of surveillance within schools are unlikely to enable staff to thrive. Leaders should make the time to check in on staff regularly, be visible and approachable and adopt an approach which supports the development of staff rather than an approach which places them under regimes of surveillance.

CURRICULUM, TEACHING AND LEARNING

Central to the whole school approach is the provision of a mental health curriculum which supports the development of pupils' mental health literacy. The term mental health literacy was first introduced in 1997 by Jorm et al and is defined as 'knowledge and beliefs about mental disorders which aid their recognition, management and prevention' (Jorm et al, 1997). Through this curriculum, all pupils learn about mental health, strategies to manage their mental health and how to receive support for their mental health. This curriculum is a discrete strand of the whole curriculum and is often delivered through personal, social and health education (PSHE). The government's statutory guidance for relationships and sex education (DfE, 2019) also requires schools to include mental health content in the curriculum. This curriculum should also educate pupils about how to keep themselves safe online and how to report online abuse.

Research demonstrates that the mental health curriculum can impact positively on young people's health and well-being as well as providing them with the skills they need to manage their own mental health (Durlak et al, 2011; Goodman et al, 2015). Research also shows that the stigma associated with mental ill-health becomes apparent to people at an early age (Campos et al, 2018), but the attitudes of young people can be changed more easily than those of adults (Corrigan and Watson, 2007) and therefore a key strand of the curriculum must focus on eradicating stigma. Chapter 3 addresses the mental health curriculum in more detail.

WORKING IN PARTNERSHIP WITH PUPILS

This strand of the whole school approach focuses on working in partnership with pupils to improve the mental health provision in the school. The emphasis on partnership positions pupils as agents of change. It enables pupils to actively contribute to the implementation of the whole school approach through various initiatives. Examples of approaches to partnership working include peer mentoring and staff–student advisory groups. More information on these approaches is provided in Chapter 4.

STAFF

A key strand of the whole school approach is staff training and development. Teachers can be supported to identify the signs of specific mental health conditions. Assessment of specific needs should always take into consideration the views of the parent(s) and the child (DfE, DoH, 2015), as well as noticing visible signs including changes in a child's mood or behaviour. A range of professional development opportunities are available to schools, including Mental Health First Aid training. A growing number of organisations now provide mental health training to schools.

Another aspect of this strand relates to staff well-being. Chapter 6 addresses this in more detail. Research demonstrates that teachers with poor mental health may feel that they are less able to support the well-being and mental health of their pupils (Sisask et al, 2014), particularly if they are struggling with their own well-being and mental health. Poor teacher well-being could therefore impact detrimentally on student well-being (Harding et al, 2019). In addition, research demonstrates that teachers who demonstrate 'presenteeism' find it more difficult to manage their classrooms effectively (Jennings and Greenberg, 2009) and are less likely to develop positive classroom and behaviour management strategies (Harding et al, 2019). Presenteeism is evident when teachers with poor well-being and mental health continue to work. The quality of their work is reduced, and this affects the quality of their relationships with their pupils (Jennings and Greenberg, 2009), pupil well-being (Harding et al, 2019) and overall teacher performance (Beck et al, 2011; Jain et al, 2013). There is an association between better teacher well-being and lower pupil psychological difficulties (Harding et al, 2019). There is also an association between lower teacher depression and better pupil well-being (Harding et al, 2019). In addition, there is an association between teacher presenteeism and pupil well-being and psychological difficulties (Harding et al, 2019). Thus, there appears to be a causal relationship between teacher and pupil mental health (Harding et al, 2019). This research highlights the importance of prioritising staff well-being as part of a whole school approach.

IDENTIFICATION AND INTERVENTION

Schools play a key role in the identification of mental health needs even though teachers are not trained health professionals. Some schools may use *universal screening* with all pupils, while others may use targeted screening with specific pupils. Screening is a systematic approach which ensures that some pupils' mental health needs do not go unnoticed. If schools rely on identifying mental ill-health through only noticing changes in a child's mood or behaviour, this may result in some needs of specific pupils being unidentified. This is because a child may not present with visible signs of mental ill-health even though they are experiencing poor mental ill-health.

Standardised surveys are available for assessing well-being, stress, resilience and life satisfaction. Examples of these are available on the Anna Freud website and are free for schools to use (see www.annafreud.org/resources/schools-and-colleges/well-being-measurement-framework-for-schools/).

Self-reporting well-being questionnaires are a useful tool to support universal screening. However, the validity of survey instruments may be compromised by a range of factors, including how pupils feel at the specific time they are asked to complete the surveys, and therefore it is important that a rounded assessment is made of the child's well-being. This might include your own observations of the child, and conversations with the child and their parents.

Schools are beginning to monitor more systematically students' mental health and well-being in a similar way to the monitoring of student attainment. Regular assessments of all students' well-being using published well-being surveys is one way of doing this. This can support schools in identifying trends over time. Some schools have purchased sophisticated software packages, which provide teachers with well-being profiles of individual students as well as overarching data for senior leaders who need to see variations by gender, ethnicity, special educational needs and/or disabilities, those students in receipt of pupil premium or other vulnerable students.

WORKING IN PARTNERSHIP WITH PARENTS

Working in partnership with parents makes sense because parents have knowledge of their child within informal contexts. The process of identifying mental ill-health in schools must be done in partnership with parents and the child. This is one of the key principles of the Code of Practice for Special Educational Needs and Disabilities (DfE, DoH, 2015). It should never be a surprise to a parent that their child has been identified by the school as having a probable mental health need. Once the need has been identified, it is important that school leaders meet regularly with parents to discuss progress and to identify future goals.

It is important to recognise that parents may also be experiencing mental ill-health. According to the Mental Health Foundation (2023), three times as many men as women die by suicide and men aged 40 to 49 have the highest suicide rates in the UK. Men are also less likely to access psychological therapies than women. Financial worries, particularly in the context of a cost-of-living crisis, can exacerbate parental stress and anxiety and parents who are also carers may be at risk of developing mental ill-health. School leaders may therefore need to consider how to support parents who are struggling with their own mental health. In addition, leaders may also need to provide support to parents so that they can more effectively support their child's mental health at home. Strategies for working in partnership with parents are addressed in Chapter 4.

REFERRAL

Schools must refer pupils to specialist mental health services if they have complex and enduring needs which cannot be met in school. A key aspect of the whole school approach is to ensure that there is a clear and transparent policy for managing referrals.

PREJUDICE-BASED BULLYING

Schools have a responsibility to uphold the principles of the Equality Act 2010. It is unlawful to directly or indirectly discriminate against individuals with protected characteristics. These include age, disability, gender reassignment, pregnancy, race, religion, sex and sexual orientation. Bullying is a form of direct discrimination and all schools should have clear policies and practices for addressing all forms of bullying.

LGBT+ BULLYING IN SECONDARY SCHOOLS

Stonewall's *School Report* (Bradlow et al, 2017), a study of over 3,700 lesbian, gay, bi and trans (LGBT) young people aged 11–19 across Britain, provides the evidence on bullying of young people who identify as LGBT+. The key findings from Stonewall are alarming: 45 per cent of LGBT+ students are bullied for being LGBT at school; 64 per cent of trans pupils are bullied; 86 per cent regularly hear phrases such as *'that's so gay'* or *'you're so gay'* in school and 84 per cent have self-harmed (Bradlow et al, 2017).

While the 2017 statistics suggest that there has been a reduction in homophobic bullying in comparison with Stonewall's 2012 data, more work needs to be done to ensure that all schools can meet their statutory duties outlined in the Equality Act 2010. There is a clear need to provide teachers with further training and education during their Initial Teacher Education programmes, and while they are in-service, to enable them to proactively address the needs of children and young people who identify as LGBT+.

CASE STUDY

A secondary school developed a commitment to student leadership of school mental health. Students from across the school planned and led a large conference on student mental health. The students researched topics such as depression, anxiety, self-harm, social media use and substance misuse. The students organised the conference and led the sessions and the conference was given high status. Five secondary schools across the Trust were invited to the conference.

BUILDING RESILIENCE

Being resilient is the ability to recover from adverse experiences. Some children (and staff) are more resilient than others. Children and young people need to be resilient in school and at home when they encounter difficult experiences. These include exam pressures, mastering difficult subject content, dealing with negative interactions from peers and dealing with challenging situations at home.

Resilience enables many children and young people to overcome adversity during their lives (Masten, 2001). However, resilient young people do not overcome difficult situations in isolation; they do so with support from the wider social networks to which they are connected (Roffey, 2017). A common understanding of resilience is the ability to 'bounce back' from difficult experiences (Roffey, 2017). While this is an important characteristic, resilience is a multi-dimensional construct (Luthar, 1993); it is possible to be more resilient in certain situations and less resilient in others (Roffey, 2017). In the latter situations, it is important to help pupils to transfer the resilience strategies that they have developed in one context to another.

PROMOTING POSITIVE USE OF SOCIAL MEDIA

Children and young people increasingly live their lives through technology. As digital natives they have grown up within the digital revolution. Consequently, they view technology as an essential tool which they use for a variety of purposes. Social media has now been around for at least a decade and its popularity is shared across young people and adults. Young people use Facebook, Snapchat and Instagram for various purposes, but research suggests that the use of social media is becoming increasingly private (Frith, 2017). For example, young people tend to access the technology in private spaces such as bedrooms, and the increasing popularity of instant messaging has resulted in online discussions taking place in private groups. Consequently, parents and teachers may not be aware of the online activities which take place.

TEENAGERS AND SOCIAL MEDIA

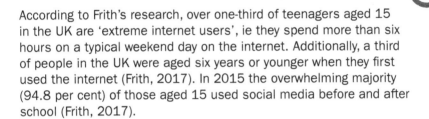

According to Frith's research, over one-third of teenagers aged 15 in the UK are 'extreme internet users', ie they spend more than six hours on a typical weekend day on the internet. Additionally, a third of people in the UK were aged six years or younger when they first used the internet (Frith, 2017). In 2015 the overwhelming majority (94.8 per cent) of those aged 15 used social media before and after school (Frith, 2017).

BENEFITS OF SOCIAL MEDIA

Social media use can support development. For example, it can facilitate access to knowledge which can have a positive impact on academic development. Young people may use social media to complete homework tasks or to clarify subject-specific misconceptions. Research suggests that young people value the social benefits of collaborating online and they may use social media for accessing specific forms of information or support (Frith, 2017). They may use social media to develop their identity as a young person. Additionally, social media can reduce social isolation for those who live long distances away from friends. It can also provide a source of support for young people through an increasing number of apps which are now available.

RISKS OF SOCIAL MEDIA

However, despite the benefits there are risks which need to be seriously considered. Lilley et al (2014) reported that online trolling was experienced by 40 per cent of their participants. Spending too much time online can create social isolation by restricting face-to-face interaction. Additionally, young people who spend too long online can experience sleep deprivation and poor sleep quality (Woods and Scott, 2016), which can then impact detrimentally on their concentration and behaviour when they are in school. The 2015 PISA research, as cited in OECD (2016), suggests that the longer people spend online, the more likely they are to experience cyberbullying, and there is evidence to suggest that social media use can impact detrimentally on children and young people's mental health, particularly for girls (Frith, 2017). Similarly, the OECD (2016) has found that excessive internet use can have a negative effect on well-being and the Office for National Statistics (2015; 2016) found that the longer people spend online, the result is a negative effect on mental health. Evidence indicates that the growth in the popularity of 'selfies' and the increasing prevalence of photoshopped images of celebrities and other idealised images of beauty results in body surveillance and lower body esteem (Frith, 2017; Tiggemann and Slater, 2014). Research has also found that girls experience a more negative mood after viewing Facebook compared to exposure to body-neutral websites (Fardouly et al, 2015). Exposure to harmful content online and the risks associated with sharing too much information with others can result in increased vulnerability. An example of this is the increase in websites which promote self-harm, resulting in its normalisation (Daine et al, 2013).

BULLYING AND SOCIAL MEDIA

Bullying through social media is different from traditional face-to-face bullying in that the harmful content is permanently available for others to see and, for the victim, this can result in repeated exposure to the content which can cause psychological distress. Additionally, the harmful content reaches a much larger audience due to the repeated sharing of that content, which can result in further psychological distress for the victim. Research demonstrates that young people are more upset by cyberbullying than exposure to online sexual content and that girls tend to be more upset about exposure to both than boys (Frith, 2017).

Responding to cyberbullying and exposure to harmful content online can be done through individuals blocking perpetrators of abuse or through parents restricting access to digital content. However, blocking access to digital content can restrict the development of digital skills (Frith, 2017) which are so vital in today's digital world. Everyone has a right to access the benefits of being online.

Developing young people's digital resilience is essential so that they are not psychologically damaged through their screen-based lifestyles. Developing a curriculum which promotes digital resilience at all key stages is one way of addressing the issues of social media bullying. All pupils should be taught about the various types of online and off-line bullying using electronic devices, and educated about the potential impacts of bullying both on perpetrators and on their victims. The proliferation of cases of high-profile individuals (for example, Members of Parliament and celebrities) who made disparaging comments online when they were younger demonstrates both the permanency of online content and the impact of such content on their professional lives as adults.

WHEN IS IT APPROPRIATE TO MAKE A REFERRAL?

CAMHS services across England are operating within a period of significant budget cuts and waiting lists are lengthy. Before you take the decision to refer a child to your local CAMHS service, it is important to be familiar with the criteria for making a referral. Although each local CAMHS service publishes its own criteria, there are some general guiding principles which you will need to consider before making a referral. These include:

+ the severity of the need;

+ the complexity of the need;

+ the duration of the need.

In relation to severity of need, you will need to consider how serious the problem is. Some problems are life-threatening or place the child at risk of harm and these will need an immediate referral. Generally, CAMHS services will only deal with cases that are severe. Examples include:

+ severe depression;

+ severe anxiety;

+ risk of suicide;

+ risk of self-harm/danger;

+ eating disorders;

+ obsessive compulsive disorders;

+ gender identity needs;

+ severe attachment needs.

This is not an exhaustive list. It merely illustrates a range of needs which may be considered to be severe. Children and young people may present other needs which you consider to be severe. In relation to severity, you will need to consider the impact of the need on the child's mental health and overall life outcomes.

You will also need to take into account the complexity of the child's need(s). Complex needs arise from multiple risk factors. Specific groups are more at risk than others of developing mental health needs. For example, children living in care or care experienced children and young people are more likely to experience mental ill-health because they may have experienced trauma. Young people who are LGBTQ+, children with disabilities and black and global majority children are also more likely to experience poor mental health. Some children are exposed to multiple risk factors which lead to complex needs.

Finally, you will need to take into account the duration of the problem. Some CAMHS services will only accept referral cases where the need has been evident for more than three months. However, judgements about whether or not a specific need is enduring need to be balanced against the potential for harm to the child. It is possible that a mental health need may be so serious that it requires immediate referral to specialist services.

In all cases where teachers or other colleagues have concerns about a child or young person, the designated safeguarding lead in the school should be informed as they are the person who will usually make the referral. The headteacher and other senior leaders may also need to be consulted. However, when making a referral it is important only to inform those people who need to know.

WHEN IS IT NOT APPROPRIATE TO MAKE A REFERRAL?

Referrals to CAMHS are not appropriate in cases where children and young people demonstrate a typical reaction to a significant life event.

These events may include:

+ parental separation;

+ bereavement of a friend or relative;

+ transition to a new school;

+ transition to a new teacher;

+ transition to a new home.

This is not an exhaustive list. It merely serves to illustrate that some needs are usual responses to traumatic or difficult situations. The child's needs can often be supported in school through pastoral support, educational psychology support or school-based counselling. The trigger for a referral will usually be when the mental health need is severe, complex and enduring. However, while some needs can subside or be met through school-based provision, it is important to remember that children will respond to similar experiences in very different ways. For example, while for some children parental separation may result in low mood, for others it may result in self-harm, severe depression or risk of suicide. Decisions about whether or not a referral is appropriate should be based not on the child's experiences, but on the impact that these experiences have had on their mental health. CAMHS will not usually take on cases where children and young people demonstrate difficulties which only occur in school, for example where a child demonstrates conduct disorder in school but where this is not evident in the home. Therefore, it is important to capture the perspectives of parents who will be able to give you additional information on the child's needs within the context of the family.

SUMMARY

A whole school approach to mental health is important because it will reduce the number of children who require mental health support in the long term. By creating a positive school culture which supports children, young people and staff, fewer will go on to develop mental health difficulties. Developing a systematic approach to universal screening reduces the likelihood that individuals will be missed. All teachers need to understand that the mental health of children and young people is their responsibility. However, the school leadership team will need to give priority to establishing positive mental health for all members of the school community. If the leadership team do not ensure that this has a strong focus, then staff are less likely to accept their responsibilities.

CHECKLIST

This chapter has addressed:

✓ the importance of a whole-school vision, supported by a set of values, which promote good mental health;

✓ the need for schools to eliminate unnecessary teacher workload;

✓ the need for schools to provide a mental health curriculum;

✓ the importance of systematically monitoring mental health provision across a school.

FURTHER READING

Howard, C, Burton, M, Levermore, D and Barrell, R (2017) *Children's Mental Health and Emotional Well-Being in Primary Schools: A Whole School Approach*. London: Sage.

Shute, R H (2016) *Mental Health and Well-being through Schools*. London: Routledge.

✛ CHAPTER 3

DESIGNING A MENTAL HEALTH CURRICULUM

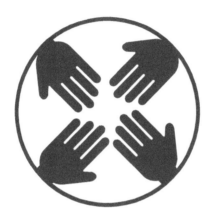

CHAPTER OBJECTIVES

By the end of this chapter, you will understand:

+ the essential components of a mental health curriculum in schools;

+ age-phase considerations in relation to curriculum design;

+ statutory guidance in relation to the school mental health curriculum.

INTRODUCTION

The curriculum is a key aspect of the whole school approach to mental health (PHE, 2021). The mental health curriculum aims to develop pupils' mental health literacy – their knowledge of mental health and their knowledge of how to access support. In addition, it also aims to eradicate the stigma that has historically been associated with mental health. This chapter provides a starting point for thinking about the curriculum content that should be included in the mental health curriculum.

WHAT IS A MENTAL HEALTH CURRICULUM?

Through a mental health curriculum, children and young people learn about the continuum of mental health. Learning about mental ill-health is one aspect of this curriculum but the curriculum is much broader in scope. Through this curriculum, children learn about how to keep mentally healthy. They will learn about the importance of physical activity, friendships and relationships and how these aspects can support good mental health. One of the aims of a mental health curriculum is to reduce the stigma about mental ill-health. Children should learn that mental health is something that everyone has and that it can fluctuate in response to everyday experiences and contexts. The curriculum should introduce young people to the stereotypes which exist in relation to mental health and directly challenge these. In addition, children should learn about resilience and how to seek support when their mental health is in decline.

DEVELOPING THE MENTAL HEALTH CURRICULUM

The mental health component of the curriculum may be taught as part of the personal, social and health education curriculum or it may be separate to this. Schools may be using a curriculum scheme that has been purchased. This is acceptable, although the scheme may need to be adapted to meet the specific needs of the pupils. If schools intend to develop their own mental health curriculum, it is useful to start by identifying the key goals of that curriculum. The questions below pro-vide a basis for identifying these goals.

CRITICAL QUESTIONS

+ What do pupils need to know and understand and be able to do in relation to mental health at the end of a specific phase of their education?

+ What are the specific mental health needs of pupils in your school?

+ How should the knowledge be sequenced so that pupils know, remember and can do more as they learn the curriculum?

The broad end goals of the mental health curriculum are sometimes referred to as *composite* knowledge. These goals should be broken down into smaller *components of knowledge* which will be taught in specific units of work and lessons. When designing the mental health curriculum, it is important to provide opportunities to revisit knowledge that has already been taught so that children do not forget the know-ledge that is stored in their long-term memory.

AN AGE-APPROPRIATE MENTAL HEALTH CURRICULUM

In designing the mental health curriculum, schools will need to decide on suitable content for pupils at specific phases of their education. Children should start learning about mental health in the early years but the content during this phase of their education typically focuses on developing children's emotional literacy. In the early years, children need to learn about the range of emotions that they will experience. These emotions include being happy, sad/upset, angry, jealous, anx-ious and excited. This is not an exhaustive list. Children need to learn about strategies to regulate their emotions and therefore through the mental health curriculum they can learn about practical things that they can do when they experience specific emotions. Many children's story books address the full spectrum of emotions that individuals experi-ence. Learning about emotions through characters in stories is a useful distancing technique because the discussions that arise are about the characters in the books rather than about individuals in the class. It is also important to challenge stereotypes in relation to emotions. Anger is not a negative emotion. It is a usual response and is something that everyone experiences. Children should not be made to feel bad for experiencing this emotion. However, they need to learn strategies for managing this emotion to prevent it from escalating.

Introducing children to the language of *mental health* from the start helps to reduce the stigma that can be associated with mental ill-health. Children should also be introduced to the language of *physical health*. They should learn about the relationship between physical and mental health and about the importance of talking to adults about their feelings.

As children progress through the mental health curriculum, they should learn about how to manage specific health conditions, including anxiety. This is particularly pertinent when pupils are undertaking public examinations or other forms of assessments. In addition, the transition from primary to secondary school is a significant transition for children and the mental health curriculum should explicitly address the transitions that children will be required to navigate during and after this critical transition. During adolescence, young people experience multiple transitions. These transitions are biological, social and psychological. Young people may also be negotiating identity transitions, particularly in relation to their gender and sexual orientation. Explicitly addressing these aspects through the mental health curriculum will reduce anxiety and support young people to realise that their emotions are typical during this phase of their lives.

CRITICAL QUESTIONS

+ What curriculum content needs to be covered in a primary mental health curriculum?

+ What curriculum content needs to be covered in the secondary mental health curriculum?

+ What curriculum content needs to be covered as pupils prepare for significant transitions? (For example, moving from primary to secondary school or moving from school to college)

EVALUATING THE IMPACT OF THE MENTAL HEALTH CURRICULUM

Impact can be evaluated through pupils knowing more, remembering more and being able to do more. One way of measuring impact is to measure pupils' mental health literacy at the start and end of the curriculum (or unit of work) using a standardised mental health literacy questionnaire. This will enable you to identify if there has been an improvement in pupils' knowledge of mental health. You might want to ascertain whether the curriculum leads to an improvement in pupils' well-being. To facilitate this, you could use a standardised well-being questionnaire before and after a curriculum intervention to identify whether there has been an improvement in their well-being score. If you are designing a series of lessons specifically to address resilience as a component of the mental health curriculum, you might use a resilience questionnaire before and after a series of lessons. Standardised questionnaires can also be sourced to measure pupils' self-esteem and confidence before and after a unit of work has been taught.

Talking to pupils about their experiences of the mental health curriculum is one of the most effective ways of evaluating the impact of the curriculum. This will enable you to find out what has worked well and any improvements which need to be made. Designing the curriculum with young people from the outset is one way of facilitating student partnership, a critical aspect of the whole school approach to mental health.

UNDERSTANDING MENTAL HEALTH

Through the mental health curriculum in primary school, children will learn that mental ill-health is only one aspect of mental health and that mental wellness (or being mentally healthy) is a critical component of mental health. Children need to be introduced to the continuum of mental health which is illustrated in Figure 3.1 and 3.2. The continuum represents the spectrum of mental health. On the very far left of the continuum is perfect mental health, while on the very far right is severe mental ill-health.

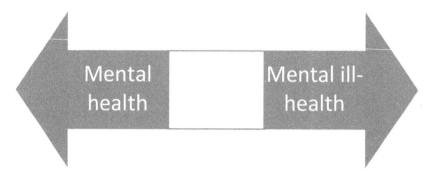

Figure 3.1. The mental health continuum

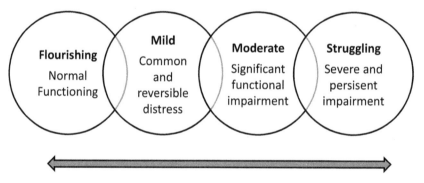

Figure 3.2. Representation of the Mental Health Continuum, adapted from published models

CRITICAL QUESTIONS

+ What factors may trigger moving from left to right across the continuum?

+ Where would you position yourself today on both models?

+ What support may people need to move from right to left on the continuum?

LEARNING ABOUT THE HISTORY OF MENTAL HEALTH

Historically, mental health has been stigmatised and people with forms of mental ill-health were once segregated from their communities and forced to live in mental health institutions. In the UK, the policy of segregating people in this way changed in the 1980s and people with mental ill-health started to receive support in their communities. Understanding the treatment of individuals with mental illnesses in the past is important because it enables young people to understand how attitudes in relation to mental health have changed. We suggest here that this could form a component of the secondary mental health curriculum, or alternatively it might be integrated into the history curriculum.

LEARNING ABOUT RESILIENCE

Resilience is an important concept for children and young people to understand because it is likely that they will experience some adversity during their lives which will impact detrimentally on their mental health. Resilience is not just an innate trait. Resilience can be enhanced by accessing social support and other forms of support. Children need to learn to be resilient in a range of situations, including being resilient in response to changing family circumstances. They also need to be resilient when they experience challenges in their friendships and relationships and in response to critical but developmental academic feedback and when they are exposed to new challenges.

Crucially, children and young people need to be resilient when they experience significant transitions. A critical transition, which can impact detrimentally on children's mental health, is the transition from primary to secondary school. During this transition, pupils also experience multiple transitions (Jindal-Snape, 2016). These include academic transitions (adapting to a new curriculum and new ways of teaching), social transitions (establishing new friendships), cultural transitions (adapting to the new environment and cultural norms of secondary school) and psychological transitions. At the time, they are also experiencing neurological transitions, changes to their bodies and some may be experiencing identity transitions. If they do not adapt to each of these various transitions, this can adversely affect their mental health and therefore teaching children about resilience in primary school, prior to this significant transition, is important. Children may also be experiencing other transitions in their daily lives. These may include parents becoming ill, parental separation, family bereavements and moving house. Children and young people will need to be resilient during these experiences because resilience will buffer the effects of transitions which are negatively experienced.

The mental health curriculum should provide children with strategies to support their resilience. These could include:

+ asking for support from adults and peers;

+ being willing to learn from mistakes;

+ investing effort in the curriculum so that they experience success;

+ keeping their long-term goals in mind to maintain motivation.

Building resilience into the mental health curriculum will provide children with the tools to 'bounce back' from negative situations and experiences. However, if children have experienced trauma, it is important to remember that it may not be possible to recover and 'bounce back' to the original state due to the long-lasting impact of trauma.

ADDRESSING STEREOTYPES AND MYTHS THROUGH THE CURRICULUM

The mental health curriculum plays a powerful role in addressing stereotypes. One of the important stereotypes that the curriculum should address is the assumption that males should not display their emotions due to the need to conform to societal gender norms. Through the curriculum, all children need to know that males can express their emotions and that this is not a sign of weakness but a sign of strength. Other myths that should be addressed through the mental health curriculum are shown below.

+ People with mental health conditions are lazy and they should just get over it!

+ People with poor mental health are dangerous or mad!

+ People with poor mental health are weak.

CRITICAL QUESTIONS

+ How would you address these stereotypes and myths in the curriculum?

+ What other stereotypes and myths exist about mental health?

STATUTORY GUIDANCE TO SUPPORT THE DESIGN OF A MENTAL HEALTH CURRICULUM

The statutory guidance for Relationships, Sex Education (RSE) and Health Education (DfE, 2019) provides you with the minimum content that needs to be addressed through the mental health curriculum.

By the end of primary school, pupils should know the following:

+ *that mental well-being is a normal part of daily life, in the same way as physical health*

+ *the benefits of physical exercise, time outdoors, community participation, voluntary and service-based activity on mental well-being and happiness;*

+ *that bullying (including cyberbullying) has a negative and often lasting impact on mental well-being;*

+ *where and how to seek support (including recognising the triggers for seeking support), including whom in school they should speak to if they are worried about their own or someone else's mental well-being or ability to control their emotions (including issues arising online);*

+ *that it is common for people to experience mental ill health. For many people who do, the problems can be resolved if the right support is made available, especially if accessed early enough;*

+ *the impact of positive and negative content online on their own and others' mental and physical well-being;*

+ *the characteristics and mental and physical benefits of an active lifestyle.*

(DfE, 2019, pp 32–3)

By the end of secondary school, pupils should know the following:

+ *how to recognise the early signs of mental well-being concerns;*

+ *common types of mental ill health;*

+ *how to critically evaluate when something they do or are involved in has a positive or negative effect on their own or others' mental health;*

+ *the benefits and importance of physical exercise, time outdoors, community participation and voluntary and service-based activities on mental well-being and happiness;*

+ *the positive associations between physical activity and promotion of mental well-being, including as an approach to combat stress;*

+ *the link between drug use, and the associated risks, including the link to serious mental health conditions;*

+ *the main changes which take place in males and females, and the implications for emotional and physical health.*

(DfE, 2019, p 42)

In addition, the statutory guidance also states:

When teaching the new subjects, schools should be aware that children may raise topics including self-harm and suicide. In talking about this content in the classroom, teachers must be aware of the risks of encouraging or making suicide seem a more viable option for pupils and avoid material being instructive rather than preventative. To avoid this, they should take care to avoid giving instructions or methods of self-harm or suicide and avoid using emotive language, videos or images.

(DfE, 2019, para 121, p 42)

LEARNING ABOUT DIGITAL SAFETY

In primary schools the mental health curriculum should also address online safety and harms. Children need to learn the rules and principles for keeping safe online, how to recognise risks, harmful content and contact, and how to report them. They need to learn about the different risks that they may be exposed to online and that the same principles apply to online relationships as to face-to-face relationships, including the importance of respect for others online, including when we are anonymous.

In secondary school, pupils need to learn about the difficulty of removing potentially compromising material placed online. They also need to learn about the negative impact of viewing pornography and the legalities associated with sharing and viewing indecent content online.

CASE STUDY

DIGITAL SAFETY

Pupils in Year 6 were learning about how to keep safe online. They discussed the importance of not sharing personal information to people they did not know, including their name, address, date of birth and the name of their school. They shared their own experiences of being online and their experiences of encountering negative content. They discussed strategies for managing this, including the importance of reporting abuse to social media platforms and the importance of telling someone about their experiences. The pupils were asked to write a guide about internet safety which could be shared with younger children in Year 4 and Year 5 to provide them with guidelines on how to keep safe online. A group of pupils volunteered to become digital champions. This was a volunteer role and the initiative was led jointly by the staff computing and mental health leaders. Pupils applied for the role and were interviewed. One of the tasks that was assigned to the digital champions was to run a workshop with parents on social media. The children had greater knowledge of social media than the parents and the purpose of the workshop was to improve parental awareness of the range of social media platforms that the children currently accessed and to provide advice to parents on how to support their child's internet use at home.

LEARNING ABOUT RELATIONSHIPS

Relationships is a key component of a mental health curriculum. Relationships, including friendships and intimate relationships, can support good mental health when they are healthy. Children and young people need to learn about the features of healthy and unhealthy relationships. This is important because unhealthy relationships, which are characterised by coercion, manipulation and control, are likely to impact negatively on mental well-being. Within this context, children also need to learn about the importance of self-respect and how this links to their own happiness. In primary schools, children need to learn about the importance of respecting others, even when they are very different from them. In the secondary curriculum, young people need to learn about consent and coercive control within relationships and strategies for reconciliation or ending relationships which are unhealthy. Pupils also need to learn about how to resist sexual pressure, sexual violence and sexual harassment within the context of relationships.

LEARNING ABOUT SUBSTANCE ABUSE

In the primary school curriculum, children need to learn about legal and illegal harmful substances and associated risks, including smoking, alcohol use and drug-taking and the relationship between substance abuse and physical and mental health. In the secondary curriculum, pupils need to learn the physical and psychological consequences of addiction, including alcohol dependency, and the associated link with serious mental health conditions and serious risks to physical health.

THE CHANGING BODY

In the primary curriculum, children need to learn about the physical and emotional changes associated with puberty and the menstrual cycle. In the secondary curriculum, pupils need to learn about the main changes which take place during adolescence and the impact of these changes on their physical and emotional health.

CASE STUDY

STRESS

In the secondary curriculum, pupils had covered curriculum content about stress. They had learned about the factors which created stress, including workload and the pressure of meeting deadlines, and that stress is a normal reaction to specific stimuli. They had understood that stress is not necessarily something that is negative. A healthy amount of stress in our lives enables us to complete tasks, work efficiently and achieve goals. The pupils had the opportunity to consider the factors which created stress in their own lives. They also had the opportunity to consider the different factors which may cause stress during the life course, for example, moving from adolescence to adulthood and the stress that individuals may encounter mid-life or in old age. The pupils were then asked to consider strategies that they used to manage stress. They created mind maps to record the strategies. Strategies included listening to music, taking a break, talking to a friend or parent, engaging in physical activity, watching a movie or taking a bath. The pupils were then asked to think about how they might recognise when the level of stress in their lives becomes too great and what they might do to counteract this.

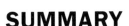

Glazzard and Szreter (2020) evaluated the efficacy of a mental health curriculum that was introduced to secondary-aged students across Cambridge, UK. A Mental Health Literacy Scale (MHLS) was used to measure students' knowledge of mental health issues pre- and post-intervention. Statistical data from these surveys were analysed using an independent samples *t*-test. Focus groups were held with students in each school, and individual semi-structured interviews were conducted with one lead teacher in each school. The data indicated that statistically significant improvements in mental health literacy were achieved, and this occurred across all genders and ethnicities. The qualitative data suggest that this programme resulted in positive attitudes towards mental health and improved knowledge of how to seek help. The data indicate that investment in similar curriculum models would be beneficial for schools in improving students' knowledge of mental health and reducing stigma.

SUMMARY

This chapter has outlined suitable content for inclusion in a school mental health curriculum. The content covered here is not exhaustive and schools need to design a curriculum that is specifically tailored to meet the needs of their pupils. The curriculum should be age-appropriate and enable pupils to know, remember and be able to do more as they learn the curriculum.

CHECKLIST

✓ The mental health curriculum is statutory in schools.

✓ Schools should design an age-appropriate mental health curriculum to develop pupils' mental health literacy.

✓ The mental health curriculum can reduce the stigma associated with mental ill-health.

FURTHER READING

Resources for primary school can be found here:
https://pshe-association.org.uk/topics/mental-health#resources-preview

Further resources to support schools in addressing mental health can be accessed using the following link:
https://educationhub.blog.gov.uk/2021/09/03/mental-health-resources-for-children-parents-carers-and-school-staff/4

✛ CHAPTER 4

WORKING IN PARTNERSHIP

CHAPTER OBJECTIVES

By the end of this chapter, you will understand:

+ effective approaches for working in partnership with parents;

+ the roles of external professionals.

INTRODUCTION

This chapter addresses the importance of working in partnership with parents, children and wider professional service teams to support children and young people's mental health. The SEND Code of Practice (DfE, DoH, 2015) highlights the importance of partnership working but it does not provide guidance on how to implement this. It is important to acknowledge that teachers are not qualified therapists. There are boundaries around their professional role and their priority is to provide education for pupils. Teachers can support the identification of mental ill-health and deliver *educational* interventions which are beneficial to children's mental health. They cannot *diagnose* mental ill-health and they cannot implement therapeutic interventions. Therefore, working in partnership with qualified professionals who can implement therapeutic interventions and who can advise teachers on strategies to implement in schools will ensure that children receive the support that they need. It is important to acknowledge, however, that there has been a lack of financial investment in mental health services, and this places children and young people at risk of not receiving timely support. This chapter also addresses these challenges.

WORKING IN PARTNERSHIP WITH PARENTS

The SEND Code of Practice (DfE, DoH, 2015) emphasises the importance of developing effective partnerships with parents. When parents and schools work together, this is significantly beneficial to the child. Parental reactions may be emotionally charged and regardless of whether the point they make is valid or not, it is crucial to allow parents to express their views and to take their concerns seriously. In nearly all instances, parents and teachers are striving for the same goals: to enable the child to flourish and to achieve the best possible outcomes. It is important to help the parent to recognise that you are both aiming for the same goals, that you care for their child and that you are doing the very best that you can for them. At the same time, it is important to demonstrate empathy towards the parent, particularly in cases where they have complex needs or face numerous challenges.

During the process of identifying mental health needs, it is important for schools to capture information about the child's well-being outside of the school. This will help you to ascertain if the mental health need is specific to the school context or whether it is evident outside of school. Any assessment of a child's needs can only be partial if it fails to capture the child's needs in a range of contexts. You may have concerns about a child. You may have noticed changes in the child's moods or behaviours. You may have recognised that the child is anxious in specific situations. You may have noticed signs that the child is self-harming. It is important to meet with parents face-to-face to discuss your concerns.

It is important to help parents understand that they have a role to play in establishing goals for their child. They should be asked to contribute to goal setting, particularly by identifying goals for their child outside of school. It is also important to help parents recognise that goals do not always have to focus on academic aspirations. Goals can relate to social, physical or emotional well-being and parents may need support in understanding how these aspects relate to mental health.

Systems should be in place to ensure that parents/carers are regularly updated on their child's progress as well as any concerns that may exist. However, effective provision goes beyond merely updating parents on their child's progress. Parents should be actively involved in helping to review their child's progress towards the identified goals. They should be invited to regular review meetings and asked to share their perspectives on their child's progress. In addition, schools could provide parents with more frequent opportunities to share their views on their child's progress.

CRITICAL QUESTIONS

+ Why might some parents be reluctant to talk about mental health with their child's school?

+ What are the potential barriers to parental partnerships and how might schools address these?

FRAMING DISCUSSIONS WITH PARENTS

The following questions or statements may be useful to help you structure an initial conversation with a parent. In this example, we have used anxiety to illustrate how to structure a conversation.

+ How are you?

+ How is George coping at home?

+ We have noticed that George becomes anxious in certain situations.

These include ...

+ Have you noticed this at home?

+ Why do you think George is anxious? Is there anything that might be causing this?

+ This is what we are doing in school to support George ... Is there anything else that we could try that might help?

+ How do you think you could support George outside of school?

+ Let's draw together a plan to support George.

PARENTAL MENTAL HEALTH

Some children and young people who have mental health needs also have parents who have mental health needs. These needs may have prevented them from forming secure attachments with their child. Additionally, in some cases where parents display mental health needs, their children may end up caring for their parent and the parent may lack the capacity to adequately care for the child. In some cases, the needs of some parents are so serious that they are unable to provide their child with a safe, caring and loving environment and in these cases schools may have no choice but to refer the matter to social care. The decision to take children into care should always be a last resort. Schools have a duty of care to ensure that children are protected from abuse and neglect. However, in many cases, parents with mental health needs can provide their child with a loving, caring, stable and nurturing environment. It is important that schools adopt a non-judgemental stance towards parents with mental health needs. Teachers and senior leaders should demonstrate empathy and kindness towards all parents, but particularly towards those who are the most vulnerable. Schools can support parents with mental health needs by signposting them to services in the community which can support them and by providing them with workshops on mental health topics.

According to Manning and Gregoire (2009), parental mental illness is associated with increased rates of mental health problems in children. Other research indicates that parents of children with an emotional disorder were more than twice as likely as other parents to have emotional disorders (NHS, 2005). Early years brain development is critical, and evidence indicates that there is a relationship between brain development and a range of outcomes, including mental and physical health (Spenrath et al, 2011). Early childhood interactions with parents and their experiences in the home influence brain development, and adverse experiences can have a negative effect on the child's mental health.

CASE STUDY

PARENT MENTAL HEALTH WORKSHOPS

One primary school had identified several parents who demonstrated signs of stress. The reasons for the stress varied across individuals but included unemployment, debt, lack of stable housing due to financial difficulties, and parents who had caring commitments to other family members. In several cases, parental stress was having a detrimental impact on the quality of the relationships with their child. Some parents were irritable, lacked patience and did not manage the behaviour of their child in a positive way. The school decided to host a workshop on stress for parents. This was led by an external provider and all parents were invited to attend. In the workshop, parents were introduced to some practical strategies to help them to manage stress more effectively. They participated well during the session and a follow-on survey indicated that parents were still using these strategies six months after participating in the workshop.

WORKING IN PARTNERSHIP WITH CHILDREN

Article 12 of the United Nations Convention on the Rights of the Child (UNCRC) states that every child has the right to express their views, feelings and wishes in all matters affecting them, and to have their views considered and taken seriously. This right applies at all times. Article 13 states that every child must be free to express their thoughts and opinions and to access all kinds of information, providing that it is within the law. The UNCRC is the most widely ratified human rights treaty in the world. The convention came into force in the UK in 1992.

According to Public Health England (2021, p 14), *'Involving students in decisions that impact on them can benefit their emotional health and well-being by helping them to feel part of the school and wider community and to have some control over their lives'*. Children and young people should be involved in the process of identifying their needs, reviewing their own progress towards goals and evaluating the efficacy of mental health interventions. They should be involved in setting their own goals and their views should be sought in relation to the content of the mental health curriculum that is being implemented by the school.

CRITICAL QUESTIONS

+ What might schools need to consider when developing models of partnership working with children and young people?

+ What other ways might schools, children and young people work in partnership to improve mental health provision?

Glazzard et al (2021) evaluated the efficacy of a peer-mentoring intervention in schools. A peer-mentoring scheme was implemented in a secondary school using a physical activity (PA) intervention to improve mental health outcomes of students who were at risk of developing mental ill-health. Older students (mentors) were matched with a group of younger students with social, emotional and mental health needs (mentees). Mentors were trained to run weekly PA sessions with their mentees and they also completed training in mental health awareness. Levels of PA increased for both mentors and mentees. Mentors reported an increase in confidence and improvements in their mental health. The mentors also acted as mental health buddies for the mentees outside the PA sessions through peer listening sessions.

CASE STUDY

MENTAL HEALTH CHAMPIONS

A secondary school introduced the role of student Mental Health Champions. Students had to apply and be interviewed for the role and not all students were accepted. Following appointment to the role, students were required to complete an intensive training course on mental health. There was an assessment at the end of this course which students were required to pass to allow them to continue in the role. Some students who did not complete the assessment were not allowed to continue in the role but were encouraged to apply in the next round.

The group met every two weeks and developed a list of priorities. One student was elected to Chair the group. Within the first 12 months, they completed the following tasks.

+ They developed a listening ear buddy scheme.

+ They worked with the Designated Senior Lead for mental health to develop the school mental health curriculum.

+ Some of the Champions took responsibility for developing a display on mental health.

+ They developed factsheets on mental health which were disseminated to all pupils. These included helpful strategies for supporting mental health and addressing exam stress.

+ They planned and ran a workshop for parents to educate them about the links between social media and mental health.

+ They reviewed the books in the library to ensure that mental health was addressed in the literature.

+ They organised a whole school mental health day, in collaboration with the Designated Senior Lead for Mental Health.

+ They were assigned a group email to enable them to provide mental health support to other pupils via email. This email account was monitored by the Designated Senior Lead for Mental Health.

+ They met with subject leaders to discuss the integration of mental health content into the subject curriculum.

+ They produced a report for Governors to document their achievements.

CRITICAL QUESTIONS

+ What safeguarding matters would need to be addressed in this case study?

+ What support might the Mental Health Champions need to enable them to carry out their roles effectively?

+ What training might the Mental Health Champions need?

THE ROLE OF THE EDUCATION MENTAL HEALTH PRACTITIONER

Following the publication of the Green Paper, *Transforming Children and Young People's Mental Health Provision* (DfE, DoH, 2017), the UK government committed to introducing Mental Health Support Teams to provide an additional layer of assistance to schools to support children and young people's mental health. The Green Paper stated:

We will fund new Mental Health Support Teams, supervised by NHS children and young people's mental health staff, to provide specific extra capacity for early intervention and ongoing help

(DfE, DoH, 2017, p 4).

These teams will be linked to groups of primary and secondary schools, and to colleges. They will provide interventions to support those with mild to moderate needs and support the promotion of good mental health and well-being. The Designated Senior Leads for Mental Health in schools will work closely with the new Support Teams, who, as part of their role, will provide a clear point of contact for schools and colleges

(DfE, DoH, 2017, p 18)

The government committed to funding to allow approximately one-fifth to one-quarter of schools to benefit from Mental Health Support Teams. This is significant because it raises a question about equity of provision. The television presenter Roman Kemp has used the platform of media to challenge the UK government to commit to additional funding so that every school can benefit from this additional layer of support.

Following the launch of this strategy in 2017, the role of the *Education Mental Health Practitioner* (EMHP) was introduced to operationalise the implementation of mental health support in schools. EMHPs must complete a postgraduate qualification which includes supervised placements with a service team. EMHPs may be responsible for implementing the following interventions:

+ providing Cognitive Behavioural Therapy (CBT) in a school/college setting for young children and adolescents showing signs of anxiety;

+ working with families;

+ delivering low-intensity clinical interventions in a school setting;

+ supporting the implementation of the whole school approach to mental health.

CRITICAL QUESTIONS

+ What are the advantages of children receiving specialist mental health support in schools rather than in hospitals or other clinical settings?

+ What are the arguments for and against the use of clinical interventions to support children's mental health?

CHILD AND ADOLESCENT MENTAL HEALTH SERVICES

Child and Adolescent Mental Health Services (CAMHS) provide specialist support for children with mental health needs. Local CAMHS services are multi-professional teams which include a range of professionals. These include psychiatrists, psychologists, social workers, nurses, support workers, occupational therapists, psychological therapists (child psychotherapists, family psychotherapists, play therapists and creative art therapists), primary mental health link workers and specialist substance misuse workers. Schools can make referrals to CAMHS, but this provision is usually reserved for young people who have severe, complex and enduring difficulties. Schools will need to check referral criteria before contacting CAMHS and any decision to refer children for support must be made with full agreement from the child's parents. Waiting times to access CAMHS services can be lengthy, and this can result in young people receiving help far too late. CAMHS does not provide support for children who have learning difficulties or behavioural problems which are evident in school, but not at home. It is a specialist service for children and young people with severe, complex and enduring mental health needs.

EDUCATIONAL PSYCHOLOGY SERVICE

Educational psychologists (EPs) may be employed by the local authority, some work individually and others are employed through private companies. The role of the EP is to provide support for children and young people who experience problems with their successful participation in school. These needs may arise due to learning difficulties or social and emotional problems. The role of an EP is multi-faceted and may include:

+ assessing learning and emotional needs through working directly with the child or young person;

+ developing and supporting therapeutic and behaviour management programmes;

+ delivering professional development for schools;

+ championing the views of parents;

+ writing reports to make formal recommendations on action to be taken, including formal Education and Health Care Plans (EHCPs);

+ attending multi-disciplinary case conferences;

+ developing and applying effective interventions to promote psychological well-being, social, emotional and behavioural development and to raise educational standards.

EPs specifically apply their knowledge of psychology to increase the participation of children and young people in their education. In cases where mental health needs start to impact on learning, behaviour and participation in education, EPs can support schools in developing specific interventions which should improve outcomes for the child. It is important that schools have comprehensive documentation to evidence what has already been done before making a referral for EP support.

This documentation should include:

+ assessments of the child in a range of contexts;

+ details about the evidence-based interventions which have been implemented to address the needs of the child;

+ evidence that the impact of interventions on outcomes for the child has been systematically monitored and evaluated;

+ evidence that the child's progress has been reviewed regularly;

+ views of the child or young person;

+ views of the parent.

Schools will need permission from the child's parents before deciding to refer a child for EP support. The EP will usually write a report and a copy is forwarded to the school and the parents. Schools should consider the recommendations which have been made by the EP and take responsibility for implementing these to secure better outcomes for the child.

SCHOOL COUNSELLING SERVICE

According to the DfE

counselling is an intervention that children or young people can voluntarily enter into if they want to explore, understand and overcome issues in their lives which may be causing them difficulty, distress and/ or confusion.

(2016, p 6)

School-based counsellors help children and young people to gain a better understanding of themselves and gain greater awareness of the personal resources they have at their disposal for managing specific situations. Providing access to a school-based counsellor provides more immediate support for a young person because there is no need to obtain a clinical diagnosis before a child can start to access school-based counselling. Schools may decide to refer a young person to school-based counselling for a variety of reasons, including where emotional and behavioural concerns exist or in cases of bullying. Students who experience academic pressure or other forms of stress may also benefit from counselling.

School-based counsellors tend to adopt a humanistic approach. This means that they tend to demonstrate unconditional positive regard for the young person, regardless of the situation, and they help them to recognise their own strengths. Some school-based counselling services operate through a 'drop-in' service or through an appointments-only system. There are strict professional boundaries between the counsellor and the client, and all counsellors should make these very clear to young people.

School-based counsellors can help young people to work towards goals and increase their resilience. They can support young people to work through relationship difficulties, manage their emotions, and increase their motivation and self-confidence. They can reduce psychological distress in young people and provide support for groups of young people that are 'at risk', including young people who identify as LGBT+ or those in care.

School-based counsellors can work with the child or young person alongside specialist support provided by CAMHs. They can also provide early intervention and suggest the need for a referral to specialist services. Some schools fund school-based counselling from pupil premium funding or from other funding streams in the school budget. School-based counsellors need a safe, private and confidential space in which to work. However, all school-based counsellors understand that confidentiality can never be absolute, especially where concerns exist about the safety and welfare of a child or young person.

SOCIAL CARE

Children's social services teams work collaboratively with schools, families and other services to ensure that children can lead safe, healthy and secure lives so that they are able to flourish. Social care services aim to protect children from abuse and neglect. They support vulnerable families in a variety of ways to ensure the best possible outcomes for children and young people.

Schools need to be vigilant and adhere to the statutory guidance in *Keeping Children Safe in Education* (DfE, 2023). Children and young people who are being abused and neglected may demonstrate signs of poor mental health. Sudden changes to moods or behaviours should be monitored carefully. If you suspect that a mental health need has been caused by abuse or neglect, then you should discuss your concerns with the designated safeguarding lead in the school and decide whether to refer the case to the Local Safeguarding Children's Board. If the child or young person is in danger, then an immediate referral should be made. Sometimes, a mental health need may not arise from abuse or neglect, but parents may require additional support in managing this need at home. In these cases, you should discuss with the parent(s) whether a referral to social care might provide an additional layer of support for the family. Some parents may become anxious about a potential referral and fear that the child will be removed from the family. You will need to reassure the parent(s) that this is extremely unlikely and will only occur if the child is in immediate danger. Separating children from their families is a last resort.

SCHOOL-BASED HEALTH SERVICES

School-based health services are delivered by qualified school nurses and health care practitioners and can provide early intervention and prevent problems from escalating. School-based health professionals can provide an additional layer of support in schools for children and young people with mental health needs. They can provide targeted intervention for a range of needs including support for managing conditions such as anxiety, depression, substance misuse or emotional health. They can provide direct education and targeted intervention on matters related to sexual health. In addition, school-based health professionals play a valuable role in enabling education colleagues to more effectively support children and young people with mental health needs through coaching or other forms of professional development.

SUMMARY

This chapter has emphasised the importance of working in partnership to support children with mental health needs. It has also highlighted strategies which schools can use to support parents with mental health needs. Parents should be provided with opportunities to participate in all decision-making processes which affect their child. The chapter has also outlined the contribution that specific professional service teams can make to supporting children and young people's mental health. We have also emphasised the importance of working in partnership with children and young people.

Young people are experts in their own lives. Therefore, if we fail to elicit their views and involve them in decisions, we lose their expert insight into the issues which they are experiencing and reduce their agency. Forward-thinking schools recognise the contribution that a student voice can make to children and young people's empowerment.

CHECKLIST

✓ Parents, children and young people should be involved in identifying goals and reviewing progress towards these.

✓ Education Mental Health Practitioners provide school-based interventions for children and young people.

✓ Referrals to CAMHS should be reserved for children and young people with the most severe mental health needs.

FURTHER READING

https://assets.publishing.service.gov.uk/media/65cb4349a7ded 0000c79e4e1/Working_together_to_safeguard_children_2023_-_ statutory_guidance.pdf
This statutory guidance on safeguarding is essential reading for all practitioners who work with children and young people.

https://participationpeople.com/how-to-implement-the-lundy-model-of-participation-across-your-organisation-a-checklist/
The Lundy Model of Participation has been adopted by many local authorities and Multi-Academy Trust to facilitate working in partnership with children and young people.

✛ CHAPTER 5

MENTAL HEALTH INTERVENTIONS IN SCHOOLS

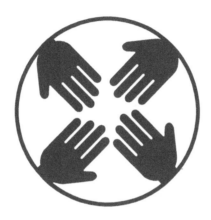

CHAPTER OBJECTIVES

By the end of this chapter, you will understand:

+ the range of mental health interventions in schools;

+ how to evaluate the effectiveness of interventions.

INTRODUCTION

This chapter outlines various mental health interventions that can be used in schools to support children's mental health and well-being. Teachers and teaching assistants are not qualified to provide forms of therapy because they are not qualified to deliver clinical interventions. Education Mental Health Practitioners are qualified to provide low-intensity interventions and CAMHS professionals can provide therapeutic interventions for children with serious and enduring mental ill-health. However, despite this, schools can implement educational interventions that will support good well-being and mental health. This chapter addresses the main interventions that can be implemented in educational contexts.

UNIVERSAL SCREENING

We have already outlined the importance of universal screening for mental health and well-being in Chapter 2 within the context of the whole school approach. A range of resources exists to support screening, including the Well-being Measurement Frameworks for Schools which can be found at: www.annafreud.org/resources/schools-and-colleges/well-being-measurement-framework-for-schools/

Children and young people do not always demonstrate observable signs of mental ill-health. Reliance on a system of identification which is based on observing changes in a child's mood or behaviour will not identify those individuals who have mental ill-health but present characteristics of healthy functioning. Toolkits such as these can support identification of needs, although it is important to recognise that children's responses on self-reporting questionnaires are only likely to reflect how they feel at the time that they complete the questions. Self-reporting questionnaires may therefore lack reliability. In addition, they may not be suitable for younger children. Training colleagues to conduct regular well-being conversations with all pupils may be more appropriate for younger children, although this is time-consuming and therefore it will require adequate resourcing. It is also important to recognise that mental health is dynamic and can fluctuate from day to day. This highlights the need for regular screening in schools.

MENTAL HEALTH EDUCATION

The importance of a mental health curriculum for all children and young people has been covered in Chapters 2 and 3. The purpose of a mental health curriculum is to reduce stigma and develop young people's mental health literacy. The term mental health literacy was first introduced in 1997 by Jorm et al; it is defined as *'knowledge and beliefs about mental disorders which aid their recognition, management and prevention'* (Jorm et al, 1997). Research shows that stigma associated with mental health problems becomes apparent to people at an early age (Campos et al, 2018), therefore the mental health curriculum plays an important role in eradicating stigma.

CASE STUDY

SECONDARY SCHOOL MENTAL HEALTH INTERVENTIONS

Pupils in Year 7 were provided with a curriculum that addressed key aspects of mental health. They learned about how to cope with stress and anxiety and the dangers of substance abuse. The community had a mental health hub which young people could access after school. It was a drop-in service and was free of charge. A representative from the hub visited the school to talk to the young people about mental health and to raise their awareness of the hub and its role in the community. Pupils completed a unit of work on stigma to help them understand the negative consequences of it and they learned about the importance of being able to reach out and ask for support.

TRAUMA-INFORMED APPROACHES

Adverse childhood experiences have a known and significant effect on children and young people's mental health. These include trauma, poor attachments with significant adults, parental alcohol and drug abuse, domestic violence, neglect and abuse (House of Commons, 2018). Trauma can result in adverse effects on brain development, cognitive functioning, attention, memory, academic performance and behaviour (Maynard et al, 2019).

73

Changes in the brain can occur in response to exposure to chronic stress and this can result in a *'fight, flight, freeze'* response (Cross et al, 2017) which can also occur in classrooms when children and young people are exposed to perceived stressors (Long, 2022). Research has demonstrated that children who have been exposed to trauma may not respond positively to traditional pastoral approaches (Baylin and Hughes, 2016) due to 'blocked trust' and a reduced ability to form social connections because of repeated abuse from adults (Baylin, 2017; Baylin and Hughes, 2016).

In England and Wales specifically, approximately a third of children and young people in schools have experienced traumatic or adverse childhood experiences such as violence, abuse or neglect (Lewis et al, 2019) and there is a limited, but growing, evidence-base on the efficacy of pastoral approaches (Long, 2022; Perfect et al, 2016; Purtle, 2020; Sparling et al, 2022).

Attachment theory and neurological evidence from psychology provides the theoretical basis for trauma-informed approaches (Long, 2022). A key emphasis within trauma-informed pedagogies is to establish positive relationships between children and adults. Relationships are the pathway through which schools can foster a sense of safety, and through which students impacted by trauma can start to regulate, connect and learn (Jacobson, 2021; Perry and Szalavitz, 2006; Perry and Winfrey, 2021). There is evidence to support the case for early relational intervention to mitigate the effects of trauma (Cross et al, 2017; Sciaraffa et al, 2017).

CASE STUDY

SOCIAL AND EMOTIONAL INTERVENTION

THREE TOWERS ALTERNATIVE PROVISION ACADEMY

Following a permanent exclusion shortly after starting at his mainstream setting, a Year 7 student was referred to Three Towers Alternative Provision (AP). The exclusion followed a series of situations where the student had displayed aggression, challenging and impulsive behaviours, and had collected items to use as weapons.

As a trauma-informed setting with experienced staff, including several accredited trauma-informed practitioners, observations were quickly made that the student was unable to access the secondary AP provision. He was on the neurodivergent pathway with highly complex needs and was in receipt of an educational health care plan (EHCP).

74

To best support the student's needs, the decision was made to integrate him into the Primary AP site to build on emotional and social skills and introduce him to the secondary setting gradually.

Three Towers applies the Thrive Approach which is carried out by accredited practitioners during interventions. Initial observations of the student led to Thrive interventions being implemented and a baseline profile for emotional needs being carried out. This suggested that the student was emotionally regulating as a 0–6 month-old. After five months of weekly Thrive interventions, his profile was revisited. Whereas the initial baseline revealed he was meeting 13 per cent of the strand criteria, he had now progressed to 52 per cent.

Following the re-profile and rapid progress, the student had a gradual reintroduction into the secondary setting. This involved a bespoke timetable, key staff and continuation of group Thrive interventions. As a result of this strategy, the student is now attending secondary full time and making good progress.

CASE STUDY

MONITORING MENTAL HEALTH AND MENTAL HEALTH INTERVENTIONS

WISTASTON ACADEMY

We are a two-form entry primary school in Cheshire with 475 pupils on roll including nursery and an alternative provision setting. We are based in an area of low socio-economic status and see the impact daily this has on children and families, with many of our children having experienced trauma. We have used various services to support our children but felt that wasn't enough.

One of our priorities is to provide a whole school approach to mental health interventions, focusing on how many children we can support and how we can ensure we provide the right interventions for our children and families in a timely way that avoids long waiting lists.

We have invested in a full-time well-being practitioner and deputy mental health lead (DMHL). Working as a team with the SENDCo and safeguarding lead, we are able to target families and children that need support by referring them to services or delivering our own evidence-based interventions in school. As well as tackling the whole school approach to mental health, the DMHL introduced a whole school survey system called Bounce Together which enables us to audit the school's mental health and well-being on a 1:1, class, year group or whole school basis, including staff. This gives us key indicators and outcomes as to where we can direct the interventions, earlier than ever before, which is so important for a Trauma-Informed Approach.

Over 300 children in the first year had support from some form of intervention. That ranged from interventions such as pet therapy, worry management, parent support, yoga or anger management. We were able to set up safe spaces in school, counselling rooms and emotion corners and all were used for various planned and unplanned interventions. When we consider that children access education better when they feel better, the investment is always worth it.

CRITICAL QUESTIONS

+ What are the dangers associated with using the word 'trauma' in schools?
+ How can trauma-informed approaches inform whole school approaches to behaviour?

MINDFULNESS

Mindfulness interventions focus on developing present-moment awareness using techniques such as breathing exercises. Some studies indicate that mindfulness can alleviate symptoms of depression and anxiety (Raes et al, 2014; Ricarte et al, 2015) and improve young people's overall sense of well-being (Lassander et al, 2021). Studies have also highlighted improvements in social skills (Schonert-Reichl and Lawlor, 2010; Viglas and Perlman, 2018) and relationships between teachers and children (Terjestam et al, 2016). However, it is important to acknowledge that there is no agreed understanding of what a school-based mindfulness intervention is and there is also a lack of research on pupils' or teachers' experiences of school-based mindfulness interventions (Abbott et al, 2024).

NURTURE GROUPS

There is evidence to suggest that where a child has not had the opportunity to form secure attachments with their carers (Bowlby, 1969;

1988), their ability to soothe themselves, regulate their emotions and form relationships has been adversely impacted (Linsell et al, 2019). Nurture groups were established by Marjorie Boxall, who worked as an educational psychologist in London in the 1960s. The theoretical underpinning for these groups is attachment theory.

According to Colley:

The nurture room sets out to provide a safe, welcoming and caring environment for learning and will replicate the home environment with a comfortable seating area, a kitchen facility for preparing food and a working area to address formal curriculum demands. A range of activities are undertaken which aim to help the young people to develop trust, communication skills and the growth of confidence and self-esteem. This might involve the sharing of news, emotional literacy sessions, turn-taking games, group activities, formal curriculum tasks or the nurture 'breakfast'.

(Colley, 2009, 291–2)

Children spend a fixed time in the nurture group setting. Emphasis is placed on developing positive relationships with adults, developing emotional and social literacy and building confidence. Sloan et al (2020) conducted an evaluation of nurture groups with a sample of 384 children, aged 5–6 years from 30 nurture group schools. The results showed clear and consistent evidence of improvements in social, emotional and behavioural outcomes for children attending nurture groups, although there was no evidence of an effect of nurture groups on the children's academic outcomes in literacy or numeracy.

CRITICAL QUESTIONS

+ What are your views on withdrawing children from their usual classrooms to enable them to participate in nurture groups?

+ What are the arguments for and against nurture groups?

PEER SUPPORT

Cross-age peer mentoring is commonly found in schools (Stapley et al, 2022), with older mentors supporting younger mentees. In the UK, there have been few robust evaluations of the efficacy of peer-mentoring interventions (Busse, Campbell and Kipping, 2018). Research in the United States has highlighted improvements in self-esteem and sense of connectedness to school (Karcher, 2005; Karcher, 2009). Although studies in the UK have reported improvements in confidence, academic performance and attitudes to learning (Messiou and Azaola, 2018; Willis, Bland, Manka and Craft, 2012), other research has also highlighted no significant impact on mentors' well-being after implementing peer-mentoring interventions (Panayiotou et al, 2020; Tymms et al, 2016). The mixed findings demonstrate that more research is required in this area.

ANTI-BULLYING INTERVENTIONS

The links between bullying and poor mental health in children and adolescents have been well established in research (for example, see Armitage, 2021). Evidence suggests that whole school approaches to reduce the prevalence of bullying are more likely to be effective than more targeted approaches (Vreeman and Carroll, 2007).

SOCIAL AND EMOTIONAL SKILLS DEVELOPMENT

Social and emotional learning (SEL) relates to the explicit development of social and emotional literacy through structured teaching which focuses on regulating emotions and social behaviours in different contexts. It also focuses on developing empathy and how to interact with others.

According to the Education Endowment Foundation (EEF):

+ *Social and emotional learning approaches have a positive impact, on average, of 4 months' additional progress in academic outcomes over the duration of an academic year.*

+ *Interventions for secondary-age pupils tend to be more effective (+5 months) than those evaluated in primary schools (+4 months).*

+ *Interventions which focus on improving social interaction tend to be more successful (+6 months) than those focusing on personal and academic outcomes (+4 months) or those aimed at preventing problematic behaviour (+5 months).*

+ *Shorter (30 mins or so) frequent sessions (4–5 times a week) appear to be the most successful structure for interventions.*

+ *Pupils from disadvantaged backgrounds are likely to have weaker SEL than more affluent peers. SEL interventions are therefore likely to support disadvantaged pupils to understand and engage in healthy relationships with peers and emotional self-regulation, both of which may subsequently increase academic attainment.*

(EEF, 2021a)

THERAPY

Educators cannot deliver therapeutic interventions because they are not clinical professionals. Therapies may include sand, Lego and art therapy, talking therapy, cognitive behavioural therapy and counselling. Many secondary schools and some primary schools operate a counselling service. Education Mental Health Practitioners may implement low-intensity clinical interventions in schools.

CASE STUDY

ART THERAPY

THREE TOWERS ALTERNATIVE PROVISION ACADEMY

A student was identified to attend therapeutic interventions following observations of challenging behaviours within the alternative provision (AP). Due to dangerous escalating behaviour both at home and school, resulting in permanent exclusion from their mainstream setting and subsequent non-attendance at a pupil referral unit, the student was then transferred to the AP. The student was observed being persistently physically aggressive and overly tactile to male peers without provocation. She was seen by many staff pulling, pushing and hitting her male peers, ignoring any staff interventions and actively encouraging others to ignore the requests and input from a senior leader. The student was unable to demonstrate any agreement to follow and comply with the AP expectations. The student was in Year 11 and impact was urgently required given the small timeframe.

The aims of the interventions were to support the student in changing behaviours and establishing positive peer and staff relationships, building self-esteem and confidence. Appropriate staff attended professional development training accredited by the British Association of Art

Therapists (BAAT.org) and applied this knowledge to focus on process art and provide positive creative experiences for the student. One-hour weekly sessions extended to three sessions over a period of several weeks. The art room became a safe space for the student to discuss the challenges she was facing each day with staff and allowed for a dialogue to be developed that encouraged her to reflect on her experiences. She was supported in emotionally regulating and making better choices.

Her attendance on arrival was 21 per cent and peaked at 92 per cent. She was able to develop positive relationships with several staff and engaged well with the majority of the subjects within her educational package. On transition from the AP, she was successful in applying for a post-16 college course.

CRITICAL QUESTIONS

+ What are the arguments for and against using therapy with children?
+ Do you think that therapeutic interventions should be implemented in schools or in clinical settings? What are the arguments for and against each?

DESIGNATED SPACES TO SUPPORT WELL-BEING

Some schools provide access to separate spaces which allow opportunities for children to decompress or self-regulate. These spaces might also be used to explicitly teach pupils the desired behaviours and practitioners might support them to develop their social and emotional regulation skills. The evidence base for social and emotional learning has already been addressed in this chapter.

SUPPORTING DISADVANTAGED PUPILS

Poverty is a significant factor in increasing the risk of individuals developing mental ill-health:

A growing body of evidence, mainly from high-income countries, has shown that there is a strong socioeconomic gradient in mental health, with people of lower socioeconomic status having a higher likelihood of developing and experiencing mental health problems. In other words, social inequalities in society are strongly linked to mental health inequalities.

(Mental Health Foundation, 2016, p 57)

Providing children and young people with a broad and rich curriculum, which enables them to develop cultural capital, will support their well-being. Restricting the curriculum is likely to adversely affect pupils' mental health. Schools should encourage pupils who are living in poverty to participate fully in a broad range of extra-curricular activities, including but not limited to access to sports. This will support social connectivity, which in turn will promote good well-being.

CASE STUDY

PRIMARY SCHOOL MENTAL HEALTH INTERVENTIONS

A primary school developed an evidence-based mental health curriculum for younger pupils. Children in the early years followed a curriculum which focused on social and emotional learning. The curriculum aimed to develop children's emotional literacy and their skills in emotional regulation. There was nurture provision for pupils in Key Stage 1 and separate nurture provision for pupils in Key Stage 2. Pupils spent part of the day in the provision to develop their social and emotional literacy and regulation skills. There was also a 'relaxation room' for pupils who needed time to decompress, staffed by a colleague who had completed a qualification in mental health.

The link between PA and well-being has long been established. Breslin et al (2016) explored connections between moderate to vigorous intensity physical activity (MVPA) and the well-being of 673 children aged 8 and 9 in Ireland from socially disadvantaged backgrounds. They found that children who participated in MVPA had higher well-being scores than those children who did not. McMahon et al (2017) concluded from their research '... *that moderately increasing activity in inactive adolescents could result in a meaningful improvement in well-being*' (p 120). Much of the recent work in this area highlights the benefits of physical activity on children's well-being (Vella et al, 2016; Tyler et al, 2016).

81

SUMMARY

This chapter has outlined the evidence base that underpins several mental health interventions that can be used with children and young people. It is critical to involve pupils and their parents or carers before interventions are implemented to ascertain the most effective interventions for individuals. It is also crucial to remember that children will respond differently to interventions and what works for one person may not work for another.

CHECKLIST

✓ The mental health curriculum aims to improve mental health literacy.

✓ Research on the efficacy of some interventions is inconclusive (for example, peer mentoring).

✓ Further research is needed to explore the efficacy of specific interventions.

FURTHER READING

Mental health interventions: www.cambridge.org/core/journals/global-mental-health/article/mental-health-provision-in-schools-approaches-and-interventions-in-10-european-countries/3386FC64E6ACE21A51F44316C5517B21

Blog: www.eif.org.uk/blog/three-reasons-why-schools-should-offer-mental-health-interventions
This is a useful article on mental health interventions in schools across ten European countries.

+ CHAPTER 6

STAFF WELL-BEING

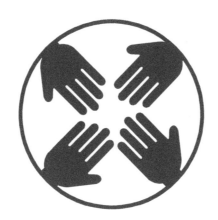

CHAPTER OBJECTIVES

By the end of this chapter, you will understand:

+ the current context of staff well-being in education;

+ how to manage your own mental health and well-being.

INTRODUCTION

Staff well-being is one strand of the whole school approach to mental health. Teacher shortage is a global problem and is therefore not specific to the UK (UNESCO, 2016). In England specifically, one of the reasons for teacher shortages is the increasing number of teachers who have decided to leave the profession, coupled with declining recruitment of pre-service teachers in initial teacher training and education. Staff shortages are resulting in a lack of availability of expert teachers across the sector and exacerbating stress levels for those who remain working in education (Ofsted, 2023). Education Support, a national charity, has demonstrated that the mental health of staff who work in the education sector is consistently declining. In 2023, the UK *Teacher Well-being Index* found that well-being in the sector is poor and continues to decline. In addition, senior leaders remain at particular risk of poor mental health (Education Support, 2023) due to the challenges of school leadership.

Despite the challenges, it is important to note that more teachers choose to remain in the profession than those who choose to leave. Teaching is a rewarding and worthwhile career and good teachers can significantly influence long-term outcomes in children and young people. The same is also true for other staff who work in education in a variety of roles. Although it is important to be aware of the challenges associated with working in education, it is also important to retain a clear sense of purpose, to recognise the impact that you make every day and to maintain an optimistic outlook.

NATIONAL CONTEXT

Data from the Teacher Well-being Index in the UK (Education Support, 2023) demonstrated a large increase in the number of teachers and senior leaders who reported that their organisational culture had a negative effect on their well-being. In addition, the research found that 78 per cent of all teachers were stressed, rising to 89 per cent for school leaders.

CRITICAL QUESTIONS

+ Why is it important to consider staff well-being?
+ What factors impact on the well-being of staff who work in education?
+ How might the factors differ for staff at different stages of their careers, for example, early career teacher, subject leader and senior leader?

MAINTAINING GOOD WELL-BEING

Well-being is a multi-dimensional dynamic construct. It includes the ability to function and thrive and an individual's sense of contentment, satisfaction and purpose in their own lives (Ruggeri et al, 2020). Physical, social, emotional, mental and spiritual dimensions of well-being interact. For example, physical and social well-being can support mental well-being because physical activity and positive social connections and relationships can support mental well-being. Mental well-being is therefore one component of overall well-being.

Figure 6.1 shows the relationship between resources and challenges. To maintain good well-being, people need to be able to access resources to help them address the challenges that they experience in their daily lives. If the challenges are high but the resources are insufficient, this can result in an imbalance which can impact negatively on an individual's well-being. When resources match the challenges, this helps to keep well-being balanced. This model highlights the importance of being able to access social, psychological and physical resources when individuals are experiencing challenges.

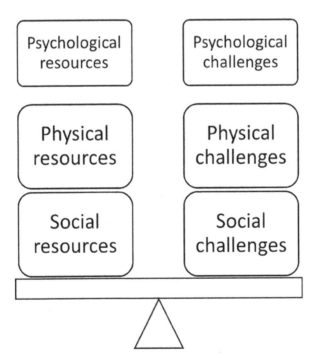

Figure 6.1. The well-being see-saw, adapted from Dodge et al (2012)

Challenges in teaching might arise from high workload or interactions with children and young people, colleagues and parents. Challenges might also arise from accountability pressures, including school inspections and pressure to maintain academic standards. To counteract these challenges, it is important to develop social networks with people that you trust so that you can talk to others about how you are feeling. Social support might be available from other colleagues in school or through people who you know outside of school, including friends, partners and other members of your family. Accessing social support will support your well-being and help you to stay resilient.

CASE STUDY

STRATEGIC LEADERSHIP OF MENTAL HEALTH

ARTHUR MELLOWS VILLAGE COLLEGE, PETERBOROUGH

Within the college, staff well-being has been a core objective since before the pandemic with a focus on workload and well-being. Since the pandemic, and as part of the work around college improvement, the designated mental health lead led an audit of staff happiness and resilience, identifying a number of concerns from staff which ranged from workload to behaviour and job satisfaction as well as praise. As part of an action plan led by this senior leader, we introduced working parties, a SWAG (Staff Well-being Action Group), a well-being survey and training for all staff. We also identified core focus areas, including workload, social events and time for connection, an understanding of mental health and well-being together with opportunities for praise from line managers and wider senior leadership.

Across the last three years, we have introduced a weekly staff bulletin which has a focus on well-being using the NHS 5 Steps programme and staff nominations to recognise the good work of colleagues. In addition, we regularly organise staff socials and events which allow for connection among colleagues. In April 2023, we ran a successful well-being action day for staff where we were able to form a partnership with a local yoga and mindfulness instructor who has continued to deliver sessions to our staff. The use of an anonymous well-being survey also allowed us to capture staff voice on key issues and create an action plan that showed staff we were listening and actioning. The training of line managers and senior leaders as well as other core staff as Mental Health First Aiders also promoted a culture of listening and support. We also allow for opportunities for Head's Commendations for staff as well as long service awards which promote praise and reinforce gratitude for our staff.

The impact of having a focus on staff well-being has greatly improved the culture of our college. Staff report their improved happiness at work via the well-being survey. This has also improved staff retention and decreased sickness absence. Utilising staff voice and involving staff in our decisions has turned well-being into everyone's responsibility, which has enabled this to be a success.

BEING RESILIENT

Resilience varies across contexts and situations. You may be more resilient in some contexts and situations and less resilient in others. In earlier literature, resilience was conceptualised as a fixed trait within individuals (Masten and Garmezy, 1985). However, in more contemporary literature, resilience is understood to be a dynamic attribute which can be enhanced through accessing resources (Luthar, 2006; Roffey, 2017; Stephens, 2013).

Definitions of resilience emphasise positive adaptation following adversity or trauma (Gayton and Lovell, 2012) and the capacity to bounce back from challenging situations and experiences (Sanderson Brewer, 2017). This ability to 'push through' regardless of circumstances is a dominant theme in the literature (Reyes et al, 2015), but this only offers a partial understanding of resilience. It is not always possible to completely bounce back from the experience of trauma and people may also need support to enable them to recover from their experiences. It is limiting, therefore, to view resilience as an innate characteristic within individuals. Resilience is not solely a trait that people do or do not possess. A person's resilience can be enhanced by access to positive social networks and relationships and workplace cultures which foster a sense of belonging, value growth and development and promote a sense of connectedness.

Figure 6.2 is a model of teacher resilience (Greenfield, 2015). It demonstrates how resilience is affected by a combination of internal and external factors.

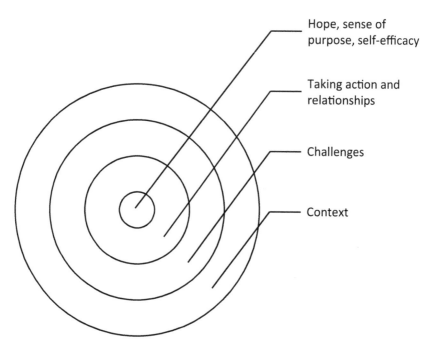

Hope, sense of
purpose, self-efficacy

Taking action and
relationships

Challenges

Context

Figure 6.2. Model of teacher resilience, adapted from Greenfield (2015)

The centre of the model identifies the *internal factors* which influence
teacher well-being. Maintaining a sense of hope and purpose can support
resilience. Having high self-efficacy can also support resilience. Teachers
with high self-efficacy are competent in their roles. Teachers with low self-
efficacy might struggle to master aspects of their roles. *Taking action*
also supports resilience. Actions might include participating in professional learning and development opportunities or making opportunities
to reflect on one's own practice. Action might also include participating
in stress-reducing activities. External factors which influence resilience
include the availability of positive social networks. Positive *relationships*
with colleagues, leaders, family, friends or children and young people
can support resilience and access to social connections are vital when
teachers are experiencing high levels of challenge. The level of *challenge*
that teachers are exposed to also influences their resilience. When
challenges are high, this can negatively impact on resilience, especially
when teachers cannot access support and resources to counteract
the challenges. When challenges are low or manageable, resilience
might be higher. Finally, the wider *context* which influences education,

including inspections, curriculum changes and public examinations and assessments, can also influence the resilience of teachers.

The model situates teacher resilience within a socio-ecological framework. It demonstrates that resilience is not solely a trait which is innate in individuals, but that access to positive social support and networks, supportive workplace cultures, manageable daily challenges and a policy context that is supportive are contributing factors which can enhance resilience in teachers. Placing the onus on individual teachers to simply increase their resilience is therefore likely to be unhelpful if these factors are not in place.

CASE STUDY

DEVELOPING A POSITIVE SCHOOL COMMUNITY

STOUR VALLEY COMMUNITY SCHOOL

What was the priority?

Our priority was to improve communication between staff and leadership and to improve the experience of both new and existing staff.

How did the school address this?

First, we wanted to assess the specific issues within our staff body so we surveyed and set up a few focus groups run by SLT and staff who were not SLT. We wanted there to be an opportunity for some people to speak directly to SLT, as well as the opportunity for all staff to feel they could be entirely honest. Once we had these responses, we knew there were specific areas we had to work on, one being communication with specific groups of staff and keeping staff up to date on changes and progress.

Secondly, SLT wanted to keep this conversation going after the initial surveys, so they introduced both a suggestions box and a 'staff shout out' box in the staffroom. These are then communicated to staff, with responses from SLT in a weekly staff bulletin. This allows staff to feel heard in an informal way, ensuring staff are aware of these comments and feedback while still allowing anonynimity. The staff shout outs also enable positive interactions to be more visible and outweigh some of the negative.

Lastly, we have assembled a staff well-being committee that meets every half term. This is chaired by a member of SLT but is an open forum to bring issues, ideas and suggestions.

What was the impact?

Positive changes have been made, staff socials have increased and it has increased and consolidated the community feeling of our school.

SELF-DETERMINATION

Self-determination theory assumes that human motivation is driven by three innate and universal psychological needs, and that personal well-being is a direct function of the satisfaction of these basic psychological needs (Deci and Ryan, 1985). These are shown in Figure 6.3.

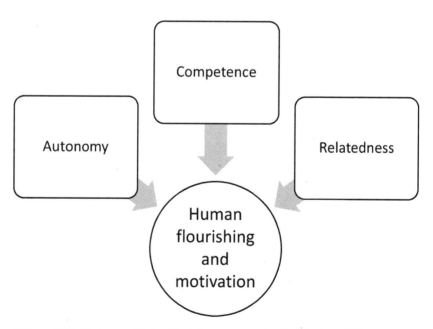

Figure 6.3. Factors which affect human motivation (adapted from Deci and Ryan, 1985)

The model is a seminal psychological theory. It assumes that autonomy, competence, and relatedness are factors which are essential for humans to flourish and be motivated. When individuals demonstrate intrinsic motivation, they are motivated by the tasks they are engaged with because they experience those tasks as interesting, challenging and rewarding. In contrast, when individuals are extrinsically motivated, they are not motivated by the tasks but by the rewards they can gain if they complete the task. Self-determination theory emphasises the role of autonomy, competence and relatedness in fostering intrinsic motivation. Most teachers enter teaching because of the satisfaction they gain from their work as educators. Although some teachers may be motivated by extrinsic rewards (for example, holidays, salary and possible promotion), the opportunity to undertake work which is interesting, intellectually challenging and deeply rewarding are the factors which promote intrinsic motivation.

Teachers are educated professionals and professional autonomy is essential to professional growth. As professionals, they need to be able to make decisions about what to teach, how to teach and how best to support their learners. The extent to which teachers have professional *autonomy* is an interesting topic of debate. Studies highlight the damaging effects of increased accountability, including inducing anxiety and fear (Nathaniel et al, 2016), fatigue and demoralisation (Buchanan, 2010), and the adverse impact on teachers' physical and mental well-being (Manning et al, 2020). The pressure to raise academic standards, government educational policies, school policies and national curriculum frameworks can restrict teacher autonomy and lead to teacher attrition. Research suggests that the teachers who remain in teaching are more likely to be working in schools with collaborative and cohesive cultures (Yonezawa et al, 2011) and supportive school leaders (Burkhauser, 2017) who value professional autonomy. In England and other countries, teaching has become a highly regulated profession. Although national policy frameworks shape the school curriculum and approaches to assessment in schools, teachers with strong and stable teacher identities can, with the support of school leaders, maintain a degree of autonomy in the classroom (Clarke, 2008). However, when autonomy is completely removed by instructing teachers about what and how to teach, this impacts negatively on their motivation and can lead to mental ill-health (Nathaniel et al, 2016).

According to Deci and Ryan (1985) *competence* also drives human motivation. Individuals can flourish when they can perform tasks and roles adequately. Self-competence (or self-efficacy) is an important component of overall self-esteem (Mruk, 1999). Individuals tend to have overall high self-esteem when they have both a positive view of themselves (self-worth) and when they can perform the tasks that are required of them (Mruk, 1999). In England, increased accountability has led to increased scrutiny. Self-competence is damaged when teachers struggle to perform their daily roles. A variety of contributory factors might impact negatively on a teacher's competence, including challenging behaviour from learners, large class sizes, insufficient resources, personal challenges and lack of support. In addition, even when teachers are competent, if they are told that they are ineffective by pupils, parents, colleagues and leaders, and subjected to constant scrutiny, this can negatively impact on their self-worth and confidence, which can subsequently impact adversely on their perceived and actual competence in the workplace.

Relatedness is the extent to which teachers can make positive social connections with colleagues, learners, parents and the school that they have chosen to work in. It is the need to interact, make connections and experience meaningful and positive relationships with others. Positive social connections increase resilience (Greenfield, 2015) and improve motivation (Deci and Ryan, 1985). Relatedness is supported when school leadership teams foster a culture of collaboration and when leaders value and trust their colleagues. Although the specific contexts of schools do influence approaches to school leadership (Towers et al, 2022), leaders who demonstrate sensitivity and empathy can make a critical difference to the ways in which teachers cope with change (Maguire et al, 2019) and experience relatedness. Leaders who *'possess a high degree of emotional intelligence'* (West-Burnham, 2009, p 13) are far better placed to buffer teachers from some of the negative effects of educational policies and foster a sense of relatedness.

CASE STUDY

STAFF WELL-BEING

THREE TOWERS ALTERNATIVE PROVISION ACADEMY

The priority was to have a focus on staff well-being as at the time a formal approach was not in place.

The audit tool within the Carnegie Centre of Excellence Mental Health Award process was used and following this, a whole school staff mental health and well-being questionnaire was established. This was in 2019 and questionnaires are now sent annually to all staff. They are anonymous and questions are consistent to monitor feedback and any changes. Results are fed back to staff and there are responses to certain feedback where actions can be taken, such as improvements within the layout of the staff room. Alongside the questionnaire, a workload review took place. Consequently, changes were made to reduce workload and policies updated. A mental health policy was created and 'well-Wednesday' was also implemented into the timetable, which, in addition to student activities, allows flexibility for staff to leave work earlier.

Feedback has consistently been overwhelmingly positive, some examples from the questionnaire being *'Three Towers makes me feel valued'*, *'there is support as soon as you walk in the building'*, *'I think we care for each other well'*. A bank of resources for staff has been created and is updated regularly. Once the formal priorities were established, additional well-being initiatives were developed such as afternoon tea boxes for all staff, staff quizzes and social activities. In 2021, Three Towers won *'most inspirational alternative provision'* at the Northwest Educate Awards, largely due to the mental health and well-being initiatives that were implemented.

CRITICAL QUESTIONS

+ What can school leaders do to foster autonomy, competence and relatedness?
+ How does school culture impact on these three factors?

CASE STUDY

MAKING WELL-BEING A PRIORITY

Leaders in a secondary school wanted to make well-being a strategic priority. To partly address this, leaders included well-being discussions in all staff appraisal/performance management review meetings. Leaders used these meetings as an opportunity to focus on well-being and asked staff to identify strategies to support their own well-being. All staff were given a target which focused on addressing their well-being. This was monitored regularly by line managers in monthly 'check in' meetings.

MANAGING WORKLOAD

In recent years, the Department for Education has provided guidance to schools to support reducing workload in schools (DfE, 2018). The school inspection framework (Ofsted, 2023) also requires school inspectors to evaluate the extent to which school leaders have taken steps to reduce workload for staff.

Reducing the time spent planning lessons is one way of managing workload. Sharing planning responsibilities between team members can also dramatically reduce workload. Using commercially produced resources (for example, published curriculum schemes) is acceptable, provided that the resources and lessons are adapted to meet the needs of learners. Some schools have a central collection of lesson plans and resources for teachers to use and adapt, thus negating the need to start planning from scratch.

Reducing the time spent marking children's work is critically important. Marking can take a substantial amount of time, and the time investment does not always lead to positive impacts on children's learning. However, evidence suggests that *feedback* (rather than marking) has a positive impact on learning (EEF, 2021b) and that although all feedback is beneficial, oral feedback is particularly effective (EEF, 2021b). Schools are now focusing more on the use of oral or live feedback within lessons. Oral feedback in lessons can be provided to learners using a variety of strategies, including sharing effective models of responses to questions, or worked examples with a whole class, using low-stakes quizzes which provide immediate feedback, providing students with individual verbal feedback, marking together as a class and peer feedback.

One approach to managing workload is to establish whether specific tasks are important and need to be completed urgently or whether they are important but not urgent and then to prioritise workload accordingly. You will also need to decide which tasks are unimportant and do not need to be completed. Important tasks are those which are necessary for enhancing pupils' learning or tasks which are largely administrative, but you are still required to complete them immediately or by a deadline. Examples of these tasks might include writing pupils' reports or inputting into data management systems. Prioritising tasks into the order in which they will be completed is a healthy working habit to adopt. Sometimes it is important to state that you do not have capacity to complete a task immediately, but that you can complete it by a certain date. This helps to manage people's expectations. Attempting to complete tasks efficiently rather than allowing tasks to build up is also a good routine to establish.

One of the challenges in teaching is to keep on top of administrative tasks such as responding to emails. Allocating specific times during the day when you check your emails is one way of addressing this, rather than checking them on multiple occasions each day.

When producing teaching resources, consider whether it is worth investing a lot of time into producing a resource that will only be used once. Consider whether you can source suitable resources from colleagues or from your online professional networks, or whether you can resource the lesson quicker.

Establishing a healthy work–life balance is important for maintaining good mental health. It is good practice to protect specific times outside of work when you do not do any work related to your job. There will always be tasks to do, and the 'to-do' list will continue to grow. To be efficient, it is impossible to complete every task to the level of perfection that you might aim for and it is rarely necessary to do so. On most occasions, it is acceptable to complete a job to a satisfactory standard rather than aiming for perfection. You will need to learn to accept that you may not complete every task that is on your list and that some tasks will need to be completed on another day.

CRITICAL QUESTIONS

+ How do you prioritise and manage your own workload? What strategies do you find effective?

+ Which tasks might be urgent in teaching? Which might be less urgent?

CASE STUDY

EXTERNAL PROFESSIONAL SUPERVISION

A large primary school invested in external professional supervision to support the well-being of staff undertaking specific roles. External professional supervision is mandatory in some professions but not in education. Staff meet with an external professional on a regular basis to talk about their work, the challenges that they experience in their roles and the decisions that they make daily. The professional supervision session is unrelated to performance management processes and sessions are confidential. This enables staff to talk openly about their work, receive professional debriefing and to jointly identify solutions to problems and next steps. The leadership team identified that staff undertaking a pastoral role, the special educational needs coordinator and the designated safeguarding lead would benefit from regular external professional supervision sessions. These staff were selected because of the nature of their roles. These colleagues were working directly with children with social, emotional and mental health needs, families and other professional services, including health and social care. Some of these colleagues were experiencing secondary trauma due to their repeated exposure to the trauma that was affecting children and families. The sessions were carefully structured and provided opportunities for debriefing. Some colleagues were personally affected by the circumstances which were adversely impacting on children and families. They found that they frequently had to offer advice to children and parents and the opportunity to talk this through with the external supervisor was extremely useful. The external supervisor was skilled in supporting the colleagues to draw boundaries between their professional and personal lives so that they could distance themselves from their work.

There is a growing body of literature outlining possible factors which influence teacher attrition (Nguyen et al, 2020). These include facets of the teacher themselves (personal factors), their students (social factors) and the school (environmental factors) (Chambers et al, 2019). Factors that can reduce attrition from teaching include seeking help from colleagues (Tait, 2008), positive school climates (Cohen et al, 2009) and role stability (Billingsley, 2004). In addition, psychosocial factors, such as teachers' emotional states (De Neve and Devos, 2017) and levels of stress that teachers experience (Billingsley and Bettini, 2019), can influence whether teachers choose to remain in teaching or leave the profession. Burnout and job satisfaction are factors which have been highlighted in the literature as crucial factors which can influence teacher attrition (Madigan and Kim, 2021) and both are likely to have negative consequences for individuals because they are enduring.

Burnout is a psychosocial syndrome that develops as a reaction to chronic work-related stress (Madigan and Kim, 2021) and is particularly common among teachers (Chang, 2009) due to the multiple demands placed on them throughout their working day

(McCarthy et al, 2016). The symptoms of burnout include emotional exhaustion, cynicism and reduced efficacy. It can lead to lower levels of job commitment, reduced physical and mental health (Hakanen et al, 2006) and absences from school (Kokkinos et al, 2005; Brunsting et al, 2014). Although burnout can influence job satisfaction, it has been argued that job satisfaction is a *psychological* dimension and burnout is a *physical* dimension of teacher well-being (Organization for Economic Co-operation and Development) (OECD, 2020). Being overloaded by work, having little or no freedom to make decisions and experiencing interpersonal conflict in the workplace can impact on overall job satisfaction and lead to burnout. Conversely, having positive relationships with colleagues, being treated fairly and experiencing teaching as a meaningful job can impact positively on both (Skaalvik and Skaalvik, 2018).

SUMMARY

This chapter has addressed staff well-being, an important part of the whole school approach to mental health. Staff thrive when they are valued, trusted, provided with autonomy and when they work with school leaders who nurture their professional growth. Tick-box initiatives which address staff well-being do not work if staff are expected to work within workplace cultures which damage their mental health. Issues of teacher retention and attrition can be addressed through developing positive school cultures which enable all staff to thrive.

CHECKLIST

✓ Access to social networks, positive workplace cultures and manageable daily challenge can improve teacher resilience.

✓ Professional autonomy, self-competence and positive connections with others support teacher motivation.

✓ Teaching is challenging, at times stressful and exhausting, but it is deeply rewarding on many levels.

FURTHER READING

Jerrim, J, Sims, S, Taylor, H, Allen, R (2020) How Does the Mental Health and Well-Being of Teachers Compare to Other Professions? Evidence from eleven survey datasets, *Review of Education*, 8(3): 659–89. This article compares the mental health of teachers to those in other professions.

Thom, J (2020) *Teacher Resilience: Managing stress and anxiety to thrive in the classroom*. John Catt Educational. This book provides practical tools for the reader to immediately implement in their own practice.

CHAPTER 7

VULNERABLE GROUPS AND INDIVIDUALS

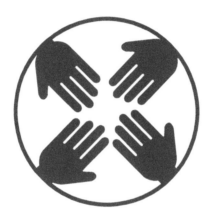

CHAPTER OBJECTIVE

By the end of this chapter, you will understand:

+ the specific mental health needs of different groups of pupils.

99

INTRODUCTION

This chapter addresses the mental health needs of specific groups of pupils. Although specific sections group children and young people into categories, it is important to recognise that all pupils are individuals. It is also important to avoid making an assumption that a child or young person will have a mental health need because they belong to a particular group. The key message in this chapter is for teachers to get to know their pupils and to work with them to find solutions to any challenges that they are experiencing.

LISTENING TO CHILDREN AND YOUNG PEOPLE

Pupils may disclose their mental health difficulties to teachers, and some will choose to disclose their personal identities. In both situations, children and young people are often seeking reassurance, understanding and affirmation. Listening to them without interrupting is a key skill that all professionals can develop. Suspending judgement, demonstrating empathy and compassion are appropriate responses and talking *with* children rather than talking *at* them is very important. Once a child or young person has made a disclosure, it is important to reflect on what needs to happen next. If you are concerned that the child is at risk of harm or if you are concerned about their welfare, then you will need to refer the case to the designated safeguarding lead. However, it is important that the child or young person understands who will be informed, what information will be communicated and what will happen next. Regularly 'checking-in' on them will mean that they know that you care and this is critical, particularly if they are not receiving support from parents or carers at home.

SUPPORTING LGBT+ CHILDREN AND YOUNG PEOPLE

Lesbian, gay, bisexual, trans, intersex, queer or questioning (LGBT+) children and young people are more likely to experience mental ill-health. Recent research shows that:

+ *LGBT+ young people are three times more likely to self-harm and twice as likely to have depression, anxiety, and panic attacks, as well as to be lonely and worry about their mental health daily;*

+ *they are more likely not to feel good about themselves daily;*

+ *they are more likely to experience an anxiety disorder;*

+ *they are more likely to contemplate suicide;*

+ *Black LGBT+ are particularly at risk of contemplating suicide;*

+ *65 per cent of disabled LGBT+ young people worry daily for their mental health.*

(Just Like Us, 2021, pp 6–7)

These statistics are supported by Mental Health First Aid England (MHFA). According to MHFA England:

+ *Mental health issues are more likely to affect young people who identify as LGBT+ than those who do not.*

+ *Young people who identify as LGBT+ are more likely to report self-harming than young people who do not identify as LGBT+.*

+ *Symptoms of depression are more common and severe in young people who identify as LGBT+ than in those who do not identify as LGBT+.*

+ *Adolescents who identify as LGBT+ are at increased risk of anxiety disorders.*

+ *11 per cent to 32 per cent of young people who identify as LGBT+ have attempted suicide in their lifetime.*

+ *Young people who identify as LGBT+ are more likely to show symptoms of eating disorders than those who do not identify as LGBT+.*

+ *People who identify as LGBT+ are at increased risk of both mental ill health and substance misuse.*

(MHFA, 2020, https://mhfaengland.org/mhfa-centre/
research-and-evaluation/mental-health-statistics/)

Meyer's Model of Minority Stress (Figure 7.1) shows the relationship between minority identities and mental ill-health.

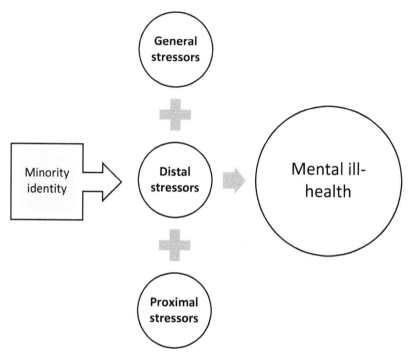

Figure 7.1. Model of minority stress (adapted from Meyer, 2003)

According to Meyer (2003) everyone is exposed to general stressors. However, individuals with a minority status are exposed to two additional stressors which can result in mental ill-health. Meyer categorised these into *distal* and *proximal* stressors. Distal stressors come from an external source but impact on the individual. Examples of distal stressors include discrimination, prejudice, bullying and harassment. Exposure to these external stressors can result in a range of mental health conditions including anxiety, depression and self-harm. Proximal stressors are internal stressors. They arise because individuals who are LGBT+, gender diverse, disabled or from global majority populations anticipate that distal stressors will occur. For individuals who are LGBT+, they may fear a negative reaction from others if their identities are disclosed and this can lead to concealment and internalised homophobia, lesbophobia, biphobia or transphobia. When this occurs, LGBT+ start to self-stigmatise by thinking that there is something wrong with them. They may be anxious about 'coming out' in case they experience negative reactions, and they may worry about accessing unsupervised social spaces, such as changing rooms, in case they experience various forms of discrimination.

Schools can address the mental health needs of LGBT+ children and young people by implementing a whole school approach to LGBT+ inclusion. One component of the whole school approach is the implementation of an LGBT+ curriculum which makes LGBT+ identities visible and fosters a culture of respect for different identities. Through this curriculum, pupils learn about the Equality Act 2010 and the protected characteristics, and they also learn how to challenge bullying if they witness it. Like the whole school approach to mental health, the whole school approach to inclusion has several components. These are shown in Figure 7.2.

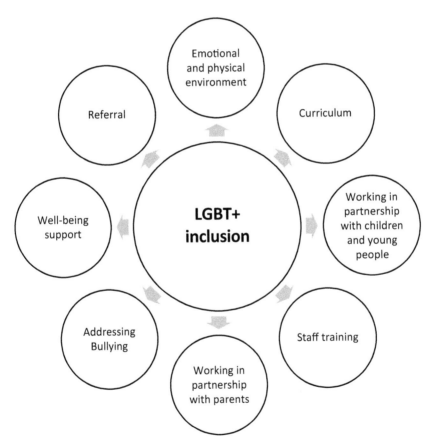

Figure 7.2. Whole school approach to LGBT+ Inclusion (adapted from Glazzard and Stones, 2019)

CRITICAL QUESTIONS

+ Based on your knowledge of the whole-school approach to mental health, which was outlined in Chapter 2, how might you address each of these aspects of the whole school approach to LGBT+ inclusion?

+ How might you adapt this model for other minority or global majority groups?

+ How might you structure a conversation with a pupil who 'comes out' to you? Write down some prompts to help you structure this conversation.

+ What is an age-appropriate LGBT+ curriculum for children and young people at different phases of their education?

SUPPORTING GENDER DIVERSE CHILDREN AND YOUNG PEOPLE

In recent years, an increasing number of children have been questioning their gender (DfE, 2023). Key terminology for teachers is summarised below.

+ **Gender questioning**: *a broad term that might describe children and young people who are questioning their biological sex and gender identity.*

+ **Social transition**: *a term often used to refer to a process by which people change their name, pronouns, clothing or use different facilities from those provided for their biological sex.*

+ **Gender incongruence**: *a medical diagnostic term for a marked and persistent incongruence between an individual's experienced gender identity and their biological sex.*

+ **Gender dysphoria**: *a similar diagnostic term to describe gender incongruence, of at least six months' duration, which is manifested by several criteria. The condition is associated with clinically significant distress or impairment in social or other important areas of functioning.*

+ **Gender identity**: *gender is a social category which may not correspond with biological sex. Gender may be male, female but it can also be a category outside of this binary.*

(Adapted from DfE, 2023, p 7)

104

The following terminology is taken from Stonewall's glossary of terms:

Trans: *an umbrella term to describe people whose gender is not the same as, or does not sit comfortably with, the sex they were assigned at birth. Trans people may describe themselves using one or more of a wide variety of terms, including (but not limited to) transgender, transsexual, gender-queer (GQ), gender-fluid, non-binary, gender-variant, crossdresser, genderless, agender, nongender, third gender, bi-gender, trans man, trans woman, trans masculine, trans feminine and neutrois.*

Transgender man: *used to describe someone who is assigned female at birth but identifies and lives as a man. This may be shortened to trans man, or FTM, an abbreviation for female-to-male.*

Transgender woman: *used to describe someone who is assigned male at birth but identifies and lives as a woman. This may be shortened to trans woman, or MTF, an abbreviation for male-to-female.*

Transphobia: *the fear or dislike of someone based on the fact they are trans, including denying their gender identity or refusing to accept it. Transphobia may be targeted at people who are, or who are perceived to be, trans.*

Transsexual: *used in the past as a more medical term (similarly to homosexual) to refer to someone whose gender is not the same as, or does not sit comfortably with, the sex they were assigned at birth. This term is still used by some although many people prefer the term trans or transgender.*

Gender reassignment: *another way of describing a person's transition. To undergo gender reassignment usually means to undergo some sort of medical intervention, but it can also mean changing names, pronouns, dressing differently and living in their self-identified gender.*

Gender expression: *how a person chooses to outwardly express their gender, within the context of societal expectations of gender. A person who does not conform to societal expectations of gender may not, however, identify as trans.*

(Stonewall, 2024, https://www.stonewall.org.uk/list-lgbtq-terms)

GUIDANCE FOR SCHOOLS

At the time of publication, the DfE non-statutory guidance, *Gender Questioning Children* (DfE, 2023), was undergoing national consultation. It is important to always put the welfare of a child or young person first and children and young people should be included in all decisions. In recent years, schools have developed a range of responses to support gender diverse children and young people, including providing gender neutral bathrooms, implementing staff training, introducing children's literature which addresses gender diversity and providing children and young people with a curriculum that addresses gender diversity.

Advice from the National Education Union (NEU) is summarised below.

+ *Do not assume you do not have any trans or non-binary students. Many trans or non-binary students are not out, and, because of a lack of knowledge of trans issues, students may not have the language to explain their feelings or identity.*

+ *Acknowledge that there will be LGBT+ and trans and non-binary people within the school community as students, parents, carers, staff and governors.*

+ *Ensure trans issues and transphobia are included within the school policy framework alongside LGBT+ equality and sex equality.*

+ *Use the curriculum and activities such as assemblies to challenge stereotypes based on sex and gender identity.*

+ *Celebrate LGBT+ History Month, Transgender Awareness Week and Transgender Day of Remembrance.*

(NEU, 2019, https://neu.org.uk/advice/equality/lgbt-equality/
supporting-trans-and-gender-questioning-students)

FRAMING A DISCUSSION WITH A GENDER-DIVERSE CHILD OR YOUNG PERSON

Use the following prompts if they disclose their gender identity to you:

+ *Ask them simply 'how can we best help you?'*

+ *Ask them if they want you to share this information with anyone else so that you can help them better in school.*

+ *Have they spoken to anyone else about their feelings or gender identity?*

+ *How do they wish to express their gender identity?*

+ *Which name and which pronouns do they use?*

(Adapted from NEU, 2019, https://neu.org.uk/advice/equality/
lgbt-equality/supporting-trans-and-gender-questioning-students)

CRITICAL QUESTIONS

+ What approach should schools take if a child or young person discloses that they are a different gender, but the parents are resistant to them changing their name, pronouns and dress?

+ How might you introduce gender diversity to children in primary schools?

+ Should schools automatically inform parents if a pupil discloses that they are a different gender? Consider the implications for both primary and secondary schools.

CASE STUDY

SUPPORTING GENDER DIVERSE YOUNG PEOPLE

Leaders in a secondary school developed a policy to support trans inclusion. The policy included clear guidance to support staff, particularly in relation to handling disclosures of gender identity. Teachers' pronouns were printed on name badges. The uniform was not gendered, and non-gendered private bathrooms were available for students who did not wish to use male or female facilities. Leaders ensured that all pupils knew that gender reassignment is a protected characteristic and transphobic bullying was explicitly addressed through the curriculum. Leaders recruited equality champions who played an important role in shaping school policies in relation to equality.

SUPPORTING REFUGEES, ASYLUM SEEKERS AND MIGRANTS

Research from the Mental Health Foundation (2024) is summarised below.

+ Asylum seekers and refugees are more likely to experience poor mental health.

+ Increased vulnerability to mental health problems is linked to both pre-migration experiences, in particular exposure to war trauma.

+ Stable settlement and social support in the host country have a positive effect on the child's psychological functioning.

SUPPORTING GLOBAL MAJORITY CHILDREN AND YOUNG PEOPLE

Minority ethnic communities in the UK are majorities in other parts of the world. Black, Asian and minority ethnic groups currently represent approximately 80 per cent of the world's population, making them the global majority. The term 'global majority' has become more popular in recent years. It refers to people who are Black, Asian, Brown, dual-heritage, indigenous to the global south and/or have been racialised as 'ethnic minorities'.

According to the Mental Health Foundation (MHF):

+ *race is not something produced by the racialised. It can be understood as having arisen from material conditions that required the delineation and organisation of people into specific groups so they could be exploited and brutalised for profit;*

+ *race and power have long been intertwined, from slavery to the legacies of colonialism, to inequalities of access and opportunity entrenched in education and health services;*

+ *racism means using the concept of race to judge or treat some people worse than others;*

+ *racism is a mental health issue because racism causes trauma;*

+ *intersectional identities can result in overlapping, concurrent forms of oppression.*

(MHF, 2023, https://www.mentalhealth.org.uk/
explore-mental-health/blogs/racism-and-mental-health)

According to the NEU:

+ *race and racism are not well understood: 'race' is a social construct, but race is mistakenly and widely used to denote difference;*

+ *racism is a structural barrier perpetuated by individuals that leads to discrimination against a person because of their race;*

+ *the majority of the people around the globe are not white and yet ideas about white superiority are still deeply influential and prevalent.*

(NEU, 2022, p 5)

Schools should have a robust anti-racist policy which outlines how racism will be addressed. Racist incidents should always be reported and addressed in line with the policy. Schools should provide an anti-racist curriculum to transform the way children and young people *think* about race, including age-appropriate content on the history of Britain, slavery, colonialism and migration. The positive contributions of Black, Asian, Brown, dual-heritage, indigenous people should be addressed in the subject curriculum and Black perspectives should be addressed throughout the year and not just in Black History Month. The NEU's framework for developing an anti-racist approach is a powerful audit tool to support schools in developing a whole school approach. Further details can be found in 'Further Reading'.

CRITICAL QUESTIONS

+ According to the NEU (2021) *'... students living in poverty are four times more likely to be permanently excluded from school than their peers'* (p 6). Why do you think this is the case?

+ Children and young people with SEND are almost six times more likely to be permanently excluded. How might you explain this?

+ Children and young people of Black African Caribbean heritage are more likely to be permanently excluded. What factors might contribute to this?

CARE EXPERIENCED CHILDREN AND CHILDREN IN CARE

Care experienced young people are not a homogeneous group. However, care experienced children and young people have consistently been found to have much higher rates of mental health difficulties (Sanders, 2020). They are approximately four times more likely to have a mental disorder than children living in their birth families (NSPCC, 2015). Research also demonstrates that carers report significant emotional and behavioural difficulties in the young people they care for (Hiller, 2020) and given that they are more likely to have experienced trauma (Sanders, 2020), this is not surprising. Most children and young people are taken into care following abuse and neglect (Sanders, 2020). Five in six children in care experience a change of home, school or social worker (NSPCC, 2015). Instability and multiple placements can re-trigger experiences of separation and loss, and mental health difficulties. Many children experience multiple moves, particularly those with significant behavioural problems (Hambrick, 2016). Children in care are often unable to access mental health support (NSPCC, 2015).

109

SUPPORTING CHILDREN WITH DISABILITIES

THE SEND Code of Practice (DfE, DoH, 2015) outlines the statutory responsibilities for schools when working with pupils with SEND. Schools are required to develop approaches for working in partnership with children and young people, parents and external agencies to best meet the needs of the child. Research demonstrates that young people with SEND are more likely to experience mental ill-health. Children and young people with SEND:

+ *are more likely to experience increased levels of anxiety;*

+ *are at greater risk for depression;*

+ *may experience higher levels of loneliness;*

+ *may have a lower self-esteem;*

+ *are at greater risk of substance abuse;*

+ *may be at greater risk of anti-social behaviour.*

www.theislandyork.org/sen-mental-health-is-there-an-increased-risk

Research has shown that a child with a learning difference is six times more likely to develop a mental health issue during their lifetime than a child without one (Emerson and Hatton, 2007). The mental health conditions might arise because of exposure to the additional proximal and distal stressors that disabled people experience (Meyer, 2003). Some mental health conditions may be linked to the disability. For example, autistic children and young people may experience anxiety and distress when there are sudden changes to routines, when they are asked to do something new for the first time or when they are exposed to specific sensory stimuli.

Schools are required to support children with disabilities using a graduated approach. This is outlined in Figure 7.3.

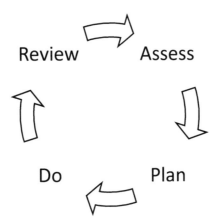

Figure 7.3. The graduated approach (DfE, DoH, 2015)

As the model shows, schools are required to carry out assessments with the child or young person to identify their needs and then use these assessments to plan specific interventions or provision for the child. These are then implemented and evaluated and the provision for the child is continually reviewed in partnership with parents, the child and external agencies. Children and young people with disabilities benefit significantly from being fully included in the full life of the school. This includes encouraging their full participation in extra-curricular activities, being included in lessons, being able to learn the same curriculum as their peers and being able to participate in the full range of educational visits. Some pupils with disabilities may benefit from specific interventions including resilience-raising interventions and all pupils with disabilities will benefit from having the opportunity to learn the full curriculum. All pupils with and without disabilities benefit from a compassionate approach to supporting behaviour where teachers respond to pupils' behaviour with empathy and work with pupils to improve their behaviour. Pupils with disabilities should be given opportunities to express their views and their opinions should be listened to, valued and acted upon where appropriate. They should be given opportunities to undertake a variety of volunteering roles in school and opportunities to contribute to setting their own goals and reviewing their own progress towards these.

YOUNG CARERS

Research cited by the Mental Health Foundation (2016) shows that caring responsibilities have been found to have a significant impact on a young carer's life, with an increased likelihood of disadvantage and health difficulties, as well as a lower likelihood of educational attainment. Children and young people may be supporting parents or elderly relatives who have conditions such as mental ill-health, other illnesses and disabilities. They may be required to support the running of the household through completing daily chores, including cooking, shopping, cleaning and providing personal care.

It is important that schools can identify these children and young people. Young carers may be balancing their family responsibilities with their education. They may be lethargic, unclean and demonstrate poor attendance and punctuality. Their academic progress may have started to decline. They may be malnourished and suffering from the effects of lack of sleep.

Concerns for the welfare of children and young people should be communicated to the designated safeguarding lead (DSL), who will then decide whether a referral to social care is necessary.

CHILDREN LIVING IN POVERTY

According to the Mental Health Foundation (2016):

+ a growing body of evidence, mainly from high-income countries, has shown that there is a strong socio-economic gradient in mental health, with people of lower socio-economic status having a higher likelihood of developing and experiencing mental health problems. In other words, social inequalities in society are strongly linked to mental health inequalities;

+ children and adults living in households in the lowest 20 per cent income bracket in Great Britain are two to three times more likely to develop mental health problems than those in the highest;

+ low income does not necessarily lead to higher rates of mental health problems, but social factors associated with lower income and socio-economic status, such as debt, can adversely affect mental health.

One of the challenges for schools is to do everything that can reasonably be expected to ensure that all pupils are attending school. Children living in poverty are particularly at risk of non-attendance. Children and young people living in poverty will benefit from a broad and rich curriculum which provides them with cultural capital. They will also benefit from participating in a wide range of extra-curricular activities, educational visits and access to free food in school.

According to the Children's Society:

Children from poorer backgrounds may not have the same opportunities as other young people their age. Many will have to work part-time jobs ... They have to work harder to overcome the obstacles that modern life puts in front of them ... Children living around debt are five times more likely to be unhappy than children from wealthier families ... More than a quarter of children from the poorest families said they had been bullied because their parents couldn't afford the cost of school.

(Children's Society, nd) www.childrenssociety.org.uk/what-we-do/our-work/ending-child-poverty/effects-of-living-in-poverty

CASE STUDY

SUPPORTING CHILDREN LIVING IN POVERTY

A primary school monitored the engagement of pupils in receipt of free school meals (FSM) and those with SEND in after-school clubs. Participation of pupils with SEND in after-school clubs was low and leaders were determined to address this. Leaders systematically sought the views of pupils and parents, and through this process they identified the need to offer some clubs at lunchtimes. Some of the pupils with SEND came to school by taxi and therefore had to leave immediately at the end of the school day. By offering activities at lunchtimes, pupils with SEND could access more enrichment activities and were therefore able to participate more fully.

Research cited by the National Education Union (NEU) (2021) demonstrates the relationship between poverty, race, ethnicity and disability:

+ young people living in more deprived areas are more likely to report lower life satisfaction than those living in less deprived areas;

+ poverty affects friendships at school with children growing up in poverty more likely to play alone and fall out with their friends, and less likely to talk to their friends about their worries;

+ black and Ethnic Minority people are overrepresented in precarious parts of the economy and are more likely to be in low-paid work. Additionally, Black and Ethnic Minority households are more likely to include larger families;

+ black and Ethnic Minority groups are not only more likely to live in poverty, which impacts detrimentally on mental health, but they are also at risk of being exposed to racism which also impacts on mental health, thus creating multiple forms of disadvantage;

+ refugees and migrants are likely to experience poverty;

+ poverty rates are especially high among families where there is a disabled child.

Children living in poverty are also more likely to be recruited into gangs so that they can generate money for their family. Once recruited, they may be asked to perform a variety of illegal activities, including drug transportation. County lines is a form of criminal exploitation. Criminals develop friendships with children and then manipulate them into drug dealing. The 'lines' refer to mobile phones that are used to control a young person who is delivering drugs, often to other towns in other counties. Young people aged 14–17 are most likely to be targeted by criminal groups, but it is not unusual for seven-year-olds to be groomed into county lines. Gradually the grooming escalates from them being initially asked to 'keep watch' to becoming drug couriers.

Schools need to be alert to signs which may indicate that children and young people are living in poverty and experiencing neglect or that they are involved in county lines. Poor appearance, poor hygiene, poor attendance and punctuality, difficulties with concentration and malnutrition could be indicators of neglect. Parents and schools also need to be alert to signs that their child might be participating in a criminal gang.

These may include the sudden appearance of a new mobile phone or multiple phones, a new style of clothing to fit in with the style of the gang, the sudden appearance of money, disengagement from usual friendships and absence from school. Any concerns should be reported to the designated safeguarding lead.

CHILDREN LIVING WITH DOMESTIC ABUSE

Domestic abuse is any incident of controlling, coercive or threatening behaviour, violence or abuse, between people in a domestic setting. Women are more likely to be victims than men (Lloyd, 2018) and the abuse can be psychological, physical, sexual, financial and emotional.

Exposure to domestic violence has a significant impact on children's mental health, with poorer educational outcomes and higher levels of mental health problems being found across the literature (Mental Health Foundation, 2016). Witnessing domestic abuse can seriously harm children and young people. According to Sterne and Poole (2010), *'although staff in schools may not be able to stop the violence at home, they are in a position to make a considerable difference to children's lives'* (p 17). Exposure to domestic abuse may result in self-blame, depression, self-harm, suicidal ideation, substance abuse, risk-taking behaviour, criminal behaviour, poor social networks, disaffection with education and eating disorders (Children's Commissioner, 2018).

Serious case reviews have repeatedly cited failure to respond to early signs of abuse, poor record keeping and sharing information too slowly as contributing to ineffective practice (Lloyd, 2018). The statutory guidance for relationships, sex and health education in England (DfE, 2019) requires schools to include domestic abuse in the curriculum. Pupils are required to learn about the signs of unhealthy and unsafe relationships and they are introduced to the principles of consent and coercion.

SUMMARY

This chapter has outlined the needs of specific groups of young people. The need to demonstrate a compassionate and empathic approach has been emphasised. Integrating social justice content into the school curriculum so that children and young people can learn about sexual orientation, gender identity, race, ethnicity, mental health and disability as part of a whole school approach to mental health increases the visibility of identities and fosters a sense of belonging. This should help to reduce the prevalence of mental ill-health.

CHECKLIST

When a child or young person discloses something:

- ✓ listen to them;
- ✓ demonstrate empathy, compassion and suspend judgement;
- ✓ talk with them, not at them;
- ✓ review the conversation and decide together if the information needs to be passed on to someone else to keep them safe. If you suspect the child or young person is at risk of harm, you must refer the case to the designated safeguarding lead;
- ✓ involve the child or young person in decisions.

FURTHER READING AND RESOURCES

www.youngminds.org.uk/professional/resources/supporting-refugee-and-asylum-seeking-children/
This video is a useful resource for supporting teachers' professional development.

https://neu.org.uk/advice/equality/race-equality
This website offers useful guidance to support schools in promoting race equality.

https://neu.org.uk/latest/library/anti-racism-charter-framework-developing-anti-racist-approach
Information about the NEUs anti-racism framework can be found using this link.

✛ CHAPTER 8

AGE-PHASE CONSIDERATIONS

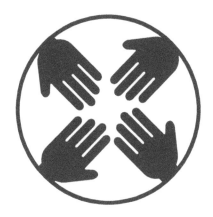

CHAPTER OBJECTIVES

By the end of this chapter, you will understand:

+ age-phase considerations in relation to mental health education;

+ the importance of supporting children and young people through transitions.

INTRODUCTION

This chapter addresses age-phase considerations in relation to mental health education in schools. During the process of designing a mental health curriculum, school leaders will need to determine what content is both *appropriate* and *relevant* to children at different phases of their education. Content which is appropriate for young people in secondary schools may not be appropriate for children in primary schools. In addition, leaders need to carefully consider the different transitions that pupils experience as they move through their education and the support that may be required at these points to help children and young people to navigate potentially difficult transitions.

MENTAL HEALTH EDUCATION IN THE EARLY YEARS

In the early years, children need to develop their emotional literacy. They need to be able to name different emotions and learn how to manage their own emotions. The transition from pre-school or nursery into school can be a significant transition for children. Most children will adapt well to this change if the systems and pedagogical approaches are similar in both settings. Children are more likely to thrive if they experience a sense of belonging and feel cared for. Rich opportunities to learn through play and positive interactions with practitioners will support their well-being. Introducing children to emotions using children's literature is a useful 'distancing' technique. This provides children with opportunities to discuss the emotions of characters in stories rather than an over-emphasis on their own behaviours. However, it is still important to support children to reflect regularly on how they are feeling, and they should be supported to discuss their emotions openly with practitioners.

Some children may find the early years environments challenging due to their sensory sensitivities. Autistic children may become distressed in response to the level of noise in the room or the social nature of the environment. Exposure to too much visual information or to certain textures (for example, sand) may also cause anxiety. It is important to remember that their behaviours (for example, stimming, screaming or head banging), although concerning, may arise because they are autistic and therefore there is a relationship between disability and mental ill-health. Strategies can be implemented to support autistic children. These include:

+ limiting exposure to bright colours by keeping colours neutral;

+ using visual timetables to provide a clear structure for the day;

+ using now and next boards so that they know what task they are currently focusing on and what task they will be doing next;

+ limiting social interaction by allowing parallel play, and gradually introducing paired and small group play;

+ establishing clear routines during the day so that they know what to expect;

+ using social stories to prepare children for unfamiliar activities.

The transition from early years settings to Key Stage 1 (ages 5–7) can also be a difficult transition. At this point, children are generally expected to sit and listen for longer periods of time, learning can become more formal with less exposure to play and the structure of the day is vastly different. Preparing children for this transition is particularly important and spending some time in their new class, prior to the transition, is one way of alleviating anxiety. Continuing with some of the pedagogical approaches that were used in the early years is also another way of reducing the 'shock effect'.

In the early years, well-designed learning environments provide opportunities for children to learn through the outdoors and to engage in physical activity. These opportunities will support children's mental health. Providing children with a broad and rich curriculum that fully addresses all areas of learning will also support good mental health.

CASE STUDY

EARLY YEARS CONSIDERATIONS

Early years leaders had identified that the transition from the early years provision to the first year of primary school was a difficult transition for many children. This transition required them to adapt to working with fewer adults, a more formal curriculum and changes to their daily routines. Leaders also had to prepare children for going into assembly and meeting much bigger children.

119

The practitioners in the early years provision worked with the Year 1 teacher to plan the transition. Children visited their new setting each week throughout the summer term, prior to changing classes in September. Parent meetings were held to inform parents about the implications of this significant transition and parents were given advice on how best to prepare their child for the transition. Some of the pedagogical approaches and routines in the Year 1 classroom were kept consistent with those in the early years setting for the first term so that the process of adaptation was gradual rather than sudden.

MENTAL HEALTH EDUCATION IN PRIMARY SCHOOLS

In primary schools, leaders need to plan the content of the mental health curriculum. During this phase of their education, children should continue to reflect on their emotions and emotional literacy and emotional regulation will still need to be embedded into the curriculum. At this stage, children start to distinguish between physical and mental health. They need to learn how to look after both aspects and they need to know that their mental health is just as important as their physical health.

In primary school, children need to learn about how to keep themselves safe online and they need to know the characteristics of healthy and unhealthy friendships. By the end of primary school, they should know:

+ *that mental well-being is a normal part of daily life, in the same way as physical health;*

+ *that there is a normal range of emotions (eg happiness, sadness, anger, fear, surprise, nervousness) and scale of emotions that all humans experience in relation to different experiences and situations;*

+ *how to recognise and talk about their emotions, including having a varied vocabulary of words to use when talking about their own and others' feelings.*

+ *how to judge whether what they are feeling and how they are behaving is appropriate and proportionate;*

+ *the benefits of physical exercise, time outdoors, community participation, voluntary and service-based activity on mental well-being and happiness;*

+ *simple self-care techniques, including the importance of rest, time spent with friends and family and the benefits of hobbies and interests;*

+ *that isolation and loneliness can affect children and that it is very important for children to discuss their feelings with an adult and seek support;*

+ *that bullying (including cyberbullying) has a negative and often lasting impact on mental well-being;*

+ *where and how to seek support (including recognising the triggers for seeking support), including to whom they should speak in school if they are worried about their own or someone else's mental well-being or ability to control their emotions (including issues arising online);*

+ *it is common for people to experience mental ill health. For many people who do, the problems can be resolved if the right support is made available, especially if accessed early enough.*

(DfE, 2019, pp 32–33)

Much of this content can be addressed through personal, social and health education using children's literature. Puppets are also an excellent resource for addressing some of this content. In Year 6, pupils may benefit from mental health support in the lead up to statutory assessment tests. Some children may experience stress and anxiety at this stage and lessons which focus on alleviating stress can be helpful. Schools should do everything they can to make statutory assessment as stress-free as possible.

CRITICAL QUESTIONS

+ Do you agree with the use of standardised testing in primary schools? What are the arguments for and against this practice?

+ What other factors may result in children experiencing anxiety in Year 6?

PRIMARY–SECONDARY TRANSITIONS

Research studies demonstrate that the transition from primary to secondary school can result in a negative impact on academic outcomes (Hopwood et al, 2016; Mudaly and Sukhdeo, 2015; Serbin et al, 2013) and lead to adverse effects on children's psychological well-being

(Jackson and Schulenberg, 2013). This transition is significant and can trigger stress and anxiety (Peters and Brooks, 2016) and lead to an increase in undesirable behaviours (Palmu et al, 2018). Research also demonstrates that children with special educational needs and/ or disabilities, such as autism, are more likely to experience difficult transitions due to increased anxiety levels associated with adapting to change (Peters and Brooks, 2016). Research also indicates that one of the effects of difficult transitions is that some young people may withdraw from formal education completely, thus potentially resulting in adverse long-term consequences (West et al, 2010).

CRITICAL QUESTIONS

+ What can schools do to prepare children for the transition from primary to secondary school?

+ What anxieties might children have prior to this transition?

+ How might these transitions affect children's mental health?

The physical change of school is only one of the transitions that occurs during primary–secondary transitions. Children also experience *academic* transitions. They are required to adapt quickly to different approaches to teaching, to new curricula and they must learn to navigate multiple subjects and teachers each day. These academic transitions contrast sharply with children's primary school education where they were largely taught by one teacher. In addition, the transition to secondary school will inevitably trigger *social transitions* for children and young people. They will meet new people and establish new friendships and previous friendships might become weakened or dissolve completely. For some, these changes will trigger *psychological transitions*, particularly if they do not feel that they fit into their new environment. Children also experience *cultural transitions*. The culture of secondary school, including learning the rules and expectations, may contrast sharply with their previous educational experience. Many children will be required, for the first time, to take responsibility for using a timetable and to arrive at different classrooms on time with the correct resources. Their relationships with teachers may be significantly different to those established with their primary school teachers. They will spend less time with them, and their teachers may not get to know them in the same way that their primary school teachers knew them. Finally, they may experience *identity transitions*. During this phase of life, it is also common for young people to explore their identities. They are gradually beginning to understand who they are and their place in the world. They may be exploring their gender identities and their sexual orientation. They may be developing a greater interest in fashion, music and other cultural interests. All these experiences will shape their sense of self and lead to a developing sense of identity.

CASE STUDY

TRANSITIONS FROM PRIMARY TO SECONDARY SCHOOL

A secondary school used a well-being scale to measure pupils' well-being on entry to the school in Year 7. The survey also focused on pupils' multiple transitions (adaptations) at this time (for example, their academic, social, cultural and psychological transitions).

Leaders systematically analysed the results to identify the average well-being score for the full cohort and the average well-being score for specific groups of pupils, including pupils with SEND. From the results, leaders could identify which transitions were smooth and which transitions were difficult for pupils. Pupils with very low scores were placed on a well-being intervention programme which was delivered by pastoral staff. These pupils also had regular 'well-being conversations' with a named member of staff. The well-being survey was repeated in Years 8, 9, 10 and 11 to capture pupils' ongoing transitions throughout secondary school.

MENTAL HEALTH IN SECONDARY SCHOOLS

Adolescence is a particularly interesting time due to the biological changes that occur in the brain. Neurons in the brain (grey matter) and synapses (junctions between neurons) are gradually pruned during adolescence. Much of the pruning takes place in the frontal lobes, specifically the frontal and parietal cortices. The volume of white matter increases and the volume of grey matter decreases. The brain continues to develop during adolescence and this development continues into early adulthood. The changes in the brain have important implications, for example, there may be a greater risk of developing addictions during adolescence. Puberty results in physical changes to the body. Hormonal changes lead to a dramatic increase in the production of testosterone in boys. These biological transitions are layered on top of the social, cultural, academic and psychological transitions that they are also navigating.

CRITICAL QUESTIONS

+ How might these biological changes influence young people's mental health?

+ What behaviours are typically demonstrated by adolescents and how are these behaviours influenced by the biological changes which are occurring?

The secondary curriculum should build on the primary curriculum to deepen children's knowledge of mental health. The curriculum should support pupils to know:

+ *how to talk about their emotions accurately and sensitively, using appropriate vocabulary;*

+ *that happiness is linked to being connected to others;*

+ *how to recognise the early signs of mental well-being concerns;*

+ *common types of mental ill health (for example, anxiety and depression);*

+ *how to critically evaluate when something they do or are involved in has a positive or negative effect on their own or others' mental health;*

+ *the benefits and importance of physical exercise, time outdoors, community participation and voluntary and service-based activities on mental well-being and happiness.*

(DfE, 2019, p 36)

In addition, pupils need to learn about online gambling, harmful behaviours online, substance abuse, the importance of quality sleep, the relationship between physical activity and mental health and the changing adolescent body and the implications of this for their mental health. Young people need to learn about the principles of consent within intimate relationships and friendships and the impact of racism, sexism, homophobia, transphobia, biphobia and disability phobia on mental health.

Older pupils can take increasing responsibility for leading on mental health, for example through peer-mentoring schemes or through the introduction of the mental health advisor role. This allows pupils to have agency and provides them with valuable opportunities to make a positive difference to their school community.

Finning et al (2022) evaluated the impact of a counselling intervention on 2,612 primary school children. Counselling is a common intervention for supporting children and young people's mental health in schools, although it is less common in primary schools than in secondary schools. The results demonstrated improvements in children's mental health, as reported by teachers and parents. Data about the children's mental health was captured after nine months of intervention and then after 21 months. This research highlights both the short- and long-term benefits of counselling as a school-based intervention.

CRITICAL QUESTIONS

+ Why do you think counselling is less commonly used in primary schools than in secondary schools?

+ Which specific group of pupils or individuals may require support from a school-based counselling service?

SUMMARY

This chapter has addressed some age-phase considerations. School mental health curricula should also address specific community issues that arise so that the curriculum reflects children and young people's lived experiences.

CHECKLIST

✓ The mental health curriculum begins in the early years.

✓ Specific mental health conditions are usually addressed in secondary education, although they can be covered in primary schools if schools determine that this is appropriate.

✓ All pupils need to know that physical health supports mental well-being.

✓ Adolescence is characterised by multiple transitions, which influence children's mental health.

FURTHER READING

Early years:
www.annafreud.org/resources/under-fives-well-being/common-difficulties/
?_gl=1*1p7a8g9*_up*MQ..&gclid=CjOKCQjw2a6wBhCVARIsABPeH1u-
ANgWpGFXMbMablgGZC-OFSViCDVe9sgttnFimE_gUSubAOfxrlsaAkewEALw_wcB

Useful guidance for working with children and young people:
www.annafreud.org/resources/children-and-young-peoples-well-being/?_gl=
1*1o1joms*_up*MQ..&gclid=CjOKCQjw2a6wBhCVARIsABPeH1u-ANgWpGF
XMbMablgGZC-OFSViCDVe9sgttnFimE_gUSubAOfxrlsaAkewEALw_wcB

Royal Society for Public Health (RSPH) (2017) *#StatusOfMind: Social Media and Young People's Mental Health and Wellbeing.* London: RSPH.

✚ CONCLUSION

WAYS FORWARD

This book has considered the role of schools in supporting children and young people's mental health. While it must be acknowledged that education professionals are not experts in health matters, schools can play an important role in promoting positive mental health. A whole school approach to mental health should reduce the numbers of young people requiring specialist provision from the health sector. Schools already play a critical role in identifying needs and providing young people with appropriate support. There are examples of best practice across the sector which need to be disseminated more widely. However, supporting children and young people in need is only part of the solution. Effective whole school approaches to mental health promote positive well-being and develop mental health literacy across all members of the school community. This book has addressed the eight principles of the whole school approach identified by Public Health England (PHE, 2021).

Mental health provision in schools is more likely to be effective when the mental health of all children, young people and staff is given high priority by the school leadership team. The government mental health strategy, *Transforming Children and Young People's Mental Health Provision* (DH/ DfE, 2017) highlights the importance of the role of schools in addressing children and young people's mental health. However, the latest Ofsted report (Ofsted, 2023) highlights several challenges that schools are currently facing. There is an increase in the number of young people who are demonstrating emotionally-based school avoidance due to anxiety. Many schools are using part-time timetables to support children with mental health needs and there is a lack of specialist mental health support from external services, resulting in delays in accessing support (Ofsted, 2023). Schools and teachers cannot take on more responsibilities and be expected to compensate for gaps in other public services. Proper investment in mental health support teams, child and adolescent mental health services and mental health hubs in every community is required to address the scale of the challenges. Teachers are not health professionals. First and foremost, they are educators. Every school should benefit from the expertise of an Education Mental Health

127

Practitioner, yet the government target falls far short of this. To address the challenges, schools cannot be expected to do more with less.

The Designated Senior Leader for Mental Health is responsible for developing universal provision for mental health, not just for children and young people in need, but for the whole school community. They are responsible for developing policies and improvement plans to support the implementation of all elements of the whole school approach outlined in this book. Additionally, all schools should demonstrate their strategic commitment to mental health by appointing a named Governor who is responsible for monitoring the quality of the mental health provision across the school. The Mental Health Governor is responsible for holding Designated Senior Leaders of Mental Health to account.

Research demonstrates that the physical, social and emotional environment in the school impacts on young people's physical, emotional and mental health and well-being as well as impacting on academic attainment (Jamal et al, 2013). In addition, research suggests that relationships between staff and students, and between students, are critical in promoting student well-being and in helping to engender a sense of belonging to the school (Cemalcilar, 2010). Key to this strand of the whole school approach is the need for schools to promote a safe environment for all members of the school community. School leaders should promote an environment which facilitates mutual respect. Policies and practices should be developed for supporting behaviour for learning, and all forms of bullying should be challenged and addressed in accordance with school policies. In addition to ensuring the safety of all members of the school community, schools should develop proactive responses by educating children and young people about bullying, discrimination and diversity to prepare young people for their responsibilities as citizens to the diverse communities in which they live. Schools should develop policies and practices which promote student voice and all adults should adopt the principle of unconditional positive regard to all children and young people.

The personal, social and emotional (PSE) curriculum in the school can impact positively on young people's health and well-being as well as providing them with the skills they need (Durlak et al, 2011; Goodman et al, 2015). A comprehensive PSE curriculum should educate young people about how to recognise and manage their feelings, how to cope with conflict and how to support others who might be in need. Schools should provide a curriculum which develops children's mental health literacy skills. This should cover a range of mental health needs including managing anxiety, stress and depression as well as more serious needs such as eating disorders. In addition, all young people should be taught to develop their resilience to adverse situations.

We believe that as well as addressing mental health content discretely, schools should embed mental health content throughout the curriculum. Subjects such as art, drama, music and English provide rich opportunities for learning about mental health. Providing children and young people with a broad, rich and relevant curriculum (including extra-curricular activities) which meets their needs is essential for promoting motivation and well-being. The physical education curriculum should provide children and young people with opportunities to participate in team sports or individual sports. These activities will allow young people to develop their resilience as well as having a positive impact on their physical, social and mental health.

According to Public Health England (2021, p 19), 'Involving students in decisions that impact on them can benefit their emotional health and wellbeing by helping them to feel part of the school and wider community and to have some control over their lives'. Schools should ensure that children and young people have appropriate channels for expressing their views. They should be consulted about curriculum, learning and teaching, and behaviour and assessment policies so that they are able to influence developments which may impact on their well-being. Schools should also provide opportunities for children and young people to form social networks, for example networks for global majority and minority groups, and monitor the impact of these networks on their well-being, attendance and academic achievements.

All staff in school should be provided with training on how to identify and support pupils with mental health needs. The Designated Senior Lead for mental health should be trained in all aspects of the whole school approach. The nominated school Governor for mental health should be provided with mental health training to develop their knowledge, skills and understanding of this complex area. Some schools are developing innovative peer-mentoring schemes where older peers support younger students with mental health needs after they have undertaken a programme of training. These schemes can develop both leadership skills and mental health literacy in peer mentors, and young people with specific needs can be supported by another young person who can offer informal support and advice.

Identification of needs in schools is often unsystematic and relies on children and young people demonstrating symptoms. Once these have been identified, the need is then targeted through intervention programmes to address the need. However, many children who have mental health needs do not demonstrate visible symptoms. This means that needs may not be identified and go unaddressed.

There are validated assessment tools which schools can adopt to support identification of needs. These include the Stirling Children's Well-being Scale and the Warwick-Edinburgh Mental Well-being Scale. These assessment tools can be given to all children and young people to provide senior leaders with a more accurate perspective on children's well-being. While these tools are primarily self-assessment tools, ie they are completed by young people, they do provide an indication of how young people are feeling at a fixed point in time. This provides leaders with school-level data which can then be interrogated by demographic information such as gender, ethnicity, disability, sexuality and age. Leaders are then able to identify trends (such as differences in well-being between groups of students and whether well-being is declining, increasing or static over time). Standardised resilience scales are also available, and these can be analysed in a similar way to well-being. Standardised tools for measuring attributes such as self-esteem and motivation can also be adopted to enable leaders to gather a whole-school perspective and to identify children and young people who require specific intervention. The impact of interventions should be systematically monitored using pre-and post-tests. Schools should adopt evidence-based interventions to address the areas of need which have been identified.

Parents, carers and the wider family play an important role in influencing children and young people's emotional health and well-being (NICE, 2013; Stewart-Brown, 2006). A whole school approach to mental health considers the various ways in which a school has the capacity to support parents through information sharing and small-group support. Schools can develop mental health literacy in parents so that parents are able to identify mental health needs in their children and provide targeted support where necessary. In addition, schools can also sign-post parents with mental health needs to appropriate services so that they get the help they need more quickly. Schools can also provide workshops to parents on a range of themes including anger management, behaviour management and domestic abuse. Effective schools have always worked in partnership with parents to secure the best possible outcomes for children and young people. Involving parents in setting targets for the young person, reviewing progress and providing support at home will foster greater parental participation.

Delays in identifying and meeting emotional and mental health needs can have detrimental effects on all aspects of children and young people's lives, including their chances of reaching their potential and leading happy and healthy lives as adults (Children and Young People's

Mental Health Coalition, 2012). Schools should work collaboratively with other professionals to ensure that children and young people get the support they need. The school nurse can play an important role in the identification of needs and they can support the referral process where this is deemed necessary.

The Education Mental Health Practitioner is vital because these professionals are qualified to deliver low intensity clinical interventions which teachers are not allowed to implement. This ensures that children receive timely support in school. However, there has, to date, been inadequate roll out of the role and further government investment is required to ensure that all schools can benefit from this support.

This book has outlined the way forward for schools in relation to supporting children and young people's mental health. Schools now need to become skilled in tracking and monitoring children's mental health with the same rigour that they currently track and monitor academic attainment. Providing specialist input for young people with identified needs is necessary but not sufficient. Adopting a whole school approach will ensure that schools can foster positive mental health for every child and young person.

REFERENCES

Abbott P, Nixon G, Stanley I and D'Ambruoso L (2024)
A Protocol for a Critical Realist Synthesis of School Mindfulness Interventions Designed to Promote Pupils' Mental Well-being. *Frontiers in Public Health.* [online] Available at: www.frontiersin.org/journals/public-health/articles/ 10.3389/fpubh.2023.1309649/full (accessed 2 April 2024).

Aldridge, J M and McChesney, K (2018)
The Relationships Between School Climate and Adolescent Mental Health and Wellbeing: A Systematic Literature Review. *International Journal Of Educational Research*, 88: 121–45.

Armitage, R (2021)
Bullying in Children: Impact on Child Health. *BMJ Paediatrics.* [online] Available at: www.ncbi.nlm.nih.gov/pmc/articles/PMC7957129/pdf/bmjpo- 2020-000939.pdf (accessed 2 April 2024).

Barber, S, (2012)
Time to Stop Stigmatising Mental Health Problems at School. [online] Available at: www.theguardian.com/teacher-network/teacher-blog/2012/apr/ 14/mental-health-stigma-school (accessed 8 August 2018).

Baylin, J (2017)
Social Buffering and Compassionate Stories: The Neuroscience of Trust Building with Children in Care. *Australian and New Zealand Journal of Family Therapy*, 38(4): 606–12.

Baylin, J and Hughes, D (2016)
The Neurobiology of Attachment-focused Therapy: Enhancing Connection and Trust in the Treatment of Children and Adolescents. London: Ringgold, Inc.

Beck A, Crain A L, Solberg L I, Unützer J, Glasgow R E, Maciosek M V, Whitebird R (2011)
Severity of Depression and Magnitude of Productivity Loss. *The Annals of Family Medicine*, 9(4): 305–11.

Billingsley, B S (2004)
Special Education Teacher Retention and Attrition: A Critical Analysis of the Research Literature. *The Journal of Special Education*, 38: 39–55.

Billingsley, B and Bettini, E (2019)
Special Education Teacher Attrition and Retention: A Review of the Literature. *Review of Educational Research*, 89: 697–744.

Blum, R W and Libbey, H P (2004)

School Connectedness: Strengthening Health and Education Outcomes for Teenagers. *Journal of School Health*, 74(7): 231–3.

Bor, W, Dean, A J, Najman, J and Hayatbakhsh, R (2014)

Are Child and Adolescent Mental Health Problems Increasing in the 21st Century? A Systematic Review. *Australian and New Zealand Journal of Psychiatry*, 48: 606–16.

Bowlby, J (1969)

Attachment and loss: Volume I: Attachment. Attachment and loss: Volume I: Attachment (pp 1–401). London: The Hogarth Press and the Institute of Psycho-Analysis.

Bowlby, J (1988)

Developmental Psychiatry Comes of Age. *The American Journal of Psychiatry*, 145(1): 1–10.

Bradlow, J, Bartram, F and Guasp, A (2017)

School Report: The Experiences of Lesbian, Gay, Bi and Trans Young People in Britain's Schools in 2017. [online] Available at: www.stonewall.org.uk/sites/default/files/the_school_report_2017.pdf (accessed 8 August 2018).

Breslin, G, Fitzpatrick, B, Brennan, D, Shannon, S, Rafferty, R, O'Brien, W, Belton, S, Chambers, F, Haughey, T, McCullagh, D, Gormley, R and Hanna, D (2016)

Physical Activity and Well-Being of 8–9-year-old Children from Social Disadvantage: An All-Ireland Approach to Health. *Mental Health and Physical Activity*, 13: 9–14.

British Youth Council (2017)

A Body Confident Future. London: British Youth Council.

Brunsting, N C, Sreckovic, M A and Lane, K L (2014)

Special Education Teacher Burnout: A Synthesis of Research from 1979 to 2013. *Education & Treatment of Children*, 37: 681–711.

Buchanan, J (2010)

May I Be Excused? Why Teachers Leave the Profession. *Asia Pacific Journal of Education*, 30(2): 199–211.

Burkhauser, S (2017)

How Much do School Principals Matter When it Comes to Teacher Working Conditions? *Educational Evaluation and Policy Analysis*, 39(1): 126–45.

Burton, M (2014)

Children and Young People's Mental Health, in Burton, M, Pavord, E and Williams, B (eds) *An Introduction to Child and Adolescent Mental Health* (pp 1–38). London: Sage.

Busse, H, Campbell, R and Kipping, R (2018)

Developing a Typology of Mentoring Programmes for Young People Attending Secondary School in the United Kingdom using Qualitative Methods. *Children and Youth Services Review*, 88: 401–15.

Butcher, J (2010)

Children and Young People as Partners in Health and Well-being, in Aggleton, P, Dennison, C and Warwick, I (eds) *Promoting Health and Well-Being Through Schools* (pp 119–33). Abingdon: Routledge.

Campos, L, Dias, P, Duarte, A, Veiga, E, Camila Dias, C and Palh, F (2018)

Is It Possible to 'Find Space for Mental Health' in Young People? Effectiveness of a School-Based Mental Health Literacy Promotion Program. *International Journal of Environmental Research and Public Health*, 15(1426): 1–12.

Cemalcilar, Z (2010)

Schools as Socialisation Contexts: Understanding the Impact of School Climate Factors on Students' Sense of School Belonging. *Applied Psychology*, 59(2): 243–72.

Chambers Mack, J, Johnson, A, Jones-Rincon, A, Tsatenawa, V and Howard, K (2019)

Why Do Teachers Leave? A Comprehensive Occupational Health Study Evaluating Intent-to-Quit in Public School Teachers. *Journal of Applied Biobehavioral Research*, 24: 1–13.

Chang, M L (2009)

An Appraisal Perspective of Teacher Burnout: Examining the Emotional Work of Teachers. *Educational Psychology Review*, 21: 193–218.

Children's Commissioner (2018)

'Are they Shouting Because of me?' Voices of Children Living in Households with Domestic Abuse, Parental Substance Misuse and Mental Health Issues. London: Children's Commissioner for England.

The Children's Society (no date)

What are the effects of child poverty? Effects Of Child Poverty | The Children's Society. [online] Available at: www.childrenssociety.org.uk/what-we-do/our-work/end ing-child-poverty/effects-of-living-in-poverty (accessed 23 April 2024).

Children and Young People's Mental Health Coalition (2012)
Resilience and Results: How to Improve the Emotional and Mental Wellbeing of Children and Young People in Your School. London: Children and Young People's Mental Health Coalition.

Clarke, M L (2008)
The Ethico-Politics of Teacher Identity. *Educational Philosophy and Theory,* 41(2): 185–200.

Clausson, E and Berg, A (2008)
Family Intervention Sessions: One Useful Way to Improve School Children's Mental Health. *Journal of Family Nursing,* 14: 289–312.

Cohen, J, McCabe, L, Michelli, N M and Pickeral, T (2009)
School Climate: Research, Policy, Practice, and Teacher Education. *Teachers College Record,* 111: 180–213.

Colley, D (2009)
Nurture Groups in Secondary Schools. *Emotional and Behavioural Difficulties,* 14(4): 291–300.

Corrigan, P and Watson, A (2007)
How Children Stigmatize People with Mental Illness. *International Journal of Social Psychiatry,* 53: 526–46.

Cross, D, Fani, N, Powers, A and Bradley, B (2017)
Neurobiological Development in the Context of Childhood Trauma. *Clinical Psychology,* 24(2): 111–24.

Cushman, P, Clelland, T and Hornby, G (2011)
Health-Promoting Schools and Mental Health Issues: A Survey of New Zealand Schools. *Pastoral Care in Education,* 29: 247–60.

Daine, K, Hawton, K, Singaravelu, V, Stewart, A, Simkin, S and Montgomery P (2013)
The Power of the Web: A Systematic Review of Studies of the Influence of the Internet on Self-Harm and Suicide in Young People. PLoS ONE, 8(10): e77555. https://doi.org/10.1371/journal.pone.0077555

Danby, G and Hamilton, P (2016)
Addressing the 'Elephant in the Room'. The Role of the Primary School Practitioner in Supporting Children's Mental Well-Being. *Pastoral Care in Education,* 34(2): 90–103.

De Neve, D and Devos, G (2017)
Psychological States and Working Conditions Buffer Beginning Teachers' Intention to Leave the Job. *European Journal of Teacher Education,* 40(1): 6–27.

Deci, E L and Ryan, R M (1985)

Intrinsic Motivation and Self-Determination in Human Behavior. Berlin: Springer Science & Business Media.

Department for Education (DfE) (2014)

Mental Health and Behaviour in Schools. [online] Available at: https://assets. publishing.service.gov.uk/media/625ee6148fa8f54a8bb65ba9/Mental_ health_and_behaviour_in_schools.pdf (accessed 31 July 2024).

Department for Education (DfE) (2016)

Mental Health and Behaviour in Schools: Departmental Advice for School Staff. London: DfE.

Department for Education (DfE) (2018)

Reducing School Workload: Support and Practical Resources for Schools to Help Reduce Workload, Including the School Workload Reduction Toolkit. [online] Available at: www.gov.uk/government/collections/reducing-school-workload (accessed 2 April 2024).

Department for Education (DfE) (2019)

Relationships Education, Relationships and Sex Education (RSE) and Health Education Statutory guidance for governing bodies, proprietors, head teachers, principals, senior leadership teams, teachers. [online] Available at: https:// assets.publishing.service.gov.uk/media/62cea352e90e071e789ea9bf/ Relationships_Education_RSE_and_Health_Education.pdf (accessed 2 April 2024).

Department for Education (DfE) (2023)

Gender Questioning Children Non-statutory Guidance for Schools and Colleges in England. London: DfE [online] Available at: https://consult.education.gov. uk/equalities-political-impartiality-anti-bullying-team/gender-questioning-child ren-proposed-guidance/supporting_documents/Gender%20Questioning%20C hildren%20%20Onnonstatutory%20guidance.pdf (accessed 2 April 2024).

Department for Education/Department of Health (DfE/DoH) (2015)

Special Educational Needs and Disability Code of Practice: 0 to 25 years – Statutory Guidance for Organisations which Work with and Support Children and Young People who Have Special Educational Needs or Disabilities. [online] Available at: https://assets.publishing.service.gov.uk/media/5a7dcb85e d915d2ac884d995/SEND_Code_of_Practice_January_2015.pdf (accessed 2 April 2024).

Department for Education/Department of Health (DfE/DoH) (2017)

Transforming Children and Young People's Mental Health Provision: A Green Paper. London: DfE/DH. Available at: https://assets.publishing.service. gov.uk/media/5a823518e5274a2e87dc1b56/Transforming_children_and_ young_people_s_mental_health_provision.pdf (accessed 2 April 2024).

Department of Health (DH) (2014)
Future in Mind: Promoting, Protecting and Improving our Children and Young People's Mental Health and Wellbeing. London: DH.

Dickins, M (2014)
A to Z of Inclusion in Early Childhood. Berkshire: Open University Press.

Dodge, R, Daly, A P, Huyton, J and Sanders, L D (2012)
The Challenge of Defining Wellbeing. *International Journal of Wellbeing,* 2(3): 222–35.

Durlak, J A, Weissberg, R, Dymnicki, A, Taylor, R and Schellinger K (2011)
The Impact of Enhancing Students' Social and Emotional Learning: A Meta-analysis of School-based Universal Interventions. *Child Development,* 82(1): 405–32.

Ecclestone, K (2014)
Stop This Educational Madness: It's Time to Resist Calls for More Mental-Health Interventions in Education. [online] Available at: www.spiked-online.com/newsite/article/stothiseducational-madness/15382#.VmtXUGcrGM8 (accessed 8 August 2019).

Ecclestone, K (2015)
Well-Being Programmes in Schools Might be Doing Children More Harm than Good. [online] Available at: http://theconversation.com/well-being-programmes-in-schools-might-be-doing-children-more-harm-than-good-36573 (accessed 8 August 2018).

Education Endowment Foundation (EEF) (2021a)
Social and Emotional Learning. [online] Available at: https://educationendowmentfoundation.org.uk/education-evidence/teaching-learning-toolkit/social-and-emotional-learning (accessed 2 April 2024).

Education Endowment Foundation (EEF) (2021b)
Teaching and Learning Toolkit. [online] Available at: https://educationendowmentfoundation.org.uk/education-evidence/teaching-learning-toolkit (accessed 2 April 2024).

Education Support (2023)
Teacher Well-Being Index 2023. London: Education Support.

Engel G L (1977)
The Need for a New Medical Model: A Challenge for Biomedicine. *Science,* 196(4286): 129–36.

Emerson E and Hatton C (2007)

Mental Health of Children and Adolescents with Intellectual Disabilities. *British Journal of Psychiatry*, 191: 493–9.

Fardouly, J, Diedrichs, P C, Vartanian, L and Halliwell, E (2015)

Social Comparisons on Social Media: The Impact of Facebook on Young Women's Body Image Concerns and Mood. *Body Image*, 13: 38–45.

Finning K, White J, Toth K, Golden S, Melendez-Torres G J and Ford T (2022)

Longer-term Effects of School-based Counselling in UK Primary Schools. *European Child and Adolescent Psychiatry*, 31(10): 1591–9.

Frith, E (2017)

Social Media and Children's Mental Health: A Review of the Evidence. London: Education Policy Institute.

Future in Mind (2015)

Future in Mind: Promoting, Protecting and Improving our Children and Young People's Mental Health and Wellbeing. London: Department for Health and NHS England.

Gayton, S and Lovell, G (2012)

Resilience in Ambulance Service Paramedics and Its Relationships with Well-Being and General Health. *Traumatology,* 18(1): 58–64.

Glazzard, J, Rose, A and Ogilvie, P (2021)

The Impact of Peer Mentoring on Students' Physical Activity and Mental Health. *Journal of Public Mental Health*, 20(2): 122–31.

Glazzard J and Stones, S, (2019)

Supporting LGBTQ+ Inclusion in Secondary Schools. Jonathan Glazzard and Samuel Stones.

Glazzard, J and Szreter, B (2020)

Developing Students' Mental Health Literacy through the Power of Sport. *Support for Learning,* 35: 222–51.

Glover, S, Burns, J, Butler, H and Patton, G (1998)

School Environments and the Emotional Wellbeing of Young People. *Family Matters*, 49: 11–16.

Goodman, A, Joshi, H, Nasim B and Tyler C (2015)

Social and Emotional Skills in Childhood and Their Long-term Effects on Adult Life. London: UCL.

Greenberg, M T, Weissberg, R P, O'Brien, M U, Zins, J E, Fredericks, L and Resnick, H (2003)
Enhancing School-Based Prevention and Youth Development Though Coordinated Social, Emotional, and Academic Learning. *American Psychologist*, 58: 466–74.

Greenfield, B (2015)
How Can Teacher Resilience be Protected and Promoted? *Educational and Child Psychology*, 32(4): 52–69.

Gumora, G and Arsenio, W F (2002)
Emotionality, Emotion Regulation, and School Performance in Middle School Children. *Journal of School Psychology*, 40: 395–413.

Hakanen, J J, Bakker, A B and Schaufeli, W B (2006)
Burnout and Work Engagement Among Teachers. *Journal of School Psychology*, 43(6): 495–513.

Hambrick, E P, Oppenheim-Weller, S, N'zi, A M and Taussig, H N (2016)
Mental Health Interventions for Children in Foster Care: A Systematic Review. *Children and Youth Services Review*, 70: 65–77.

Harding S, Morris R, Gunnell D, Ford T, Hollingworth W, Tilling K, Evans R, Bell S, Grey J, Brockman R, Campbell R, Araya R, Murphy S and Kidger J (2019)
Is Teachers' Mental Health and Wellbeing Associated with Students' Mental Health and Wellbeing? *Journal of Affective Disorders*, 1(242): 180–7.

Hiller R M, Halligan S L, Meiser-Stedman R, Elliott E and Rutter-Eley E (2020)
Supporting the Emotional Needs of Young People in Care: A Qualitative Study of Foster Carer Perspectives. *BMJ Open*, 10(3): e033317.

House of Commons (2018)
The Government's Green Paper on Mental Health: Failing a Generation. London: House of Commons Education and Health and Social Care Committees.

Jackson, K and Schulenberg, J (2013)
Alcohol use during the transition from Middle School to High School: National Panel Data on Prevalence and Moderators. *Developmental Psychology*, 49: 2147–58.

Jacobson, M R (2021)
An Exploratory Analysis of the Necessity and Utility of Trauma-informed Practices in Education. *Preventing School Failure*, 65(2): 124–34.

Jain, G, Roy, A, Harikrishnan, V, Yu, S, Dabbous, O and Lawrence, C (2013)

Patient-reported Depression Severity Measured by the PHQ-9 and Impact on Work Productivity: Results from a Survey of Full-time Employees in the United States. *Journal of Occupational and Environmental Medicine*, 55(3): 252–8.

Jamal, F, Fletcher, A, Harden, A, Wells, H, Thomas, J and Bonell, C (2013)

The School Environment and Student Health: A Systematic Review and Meta-Ethnography of Qualitative Research. *BMC Public Health*, 13(798): 1–11.

Jennings, P A, and Greenberg, M T (2009)

The Prosocial Classroom: Teacher Social and Emotional Competence in Relation to Student and Classroom Outcomes. *Review of Educational Research*, 79(1): 491–525.

Jindal-Snape, D (2016)

A–Z of Transitions. London: Palgrave.

Jorm, A, Korten, A, Jacomb, P, Christensen, H, Rodgers, B and Pollitt, P (1997)

'Mental Health Literacy': A Survey of the Public's Ability to Recognise Mental Disorders and their Beliefs about the Effectiveness of Treatment. *The Medical Journal of Australia*, 166: 182–6.

Just Like Us (2021)

Growing up LGBT+: The Impact of School, Home and Coronavirus on LGBT+ Young People. London: Just Like Us. [online] Available at: www.justlikeus.org/wp-content/uploads/2021/11/Just-Like-Us-2021-report-Growing-Up-LGBT.pdf (accessed 2 April 2024).

Karcher, M (2009)

Increases in Academic Connectedness and Self-esteem among High School Students who Serve as Cross-age Peer Mentors. *Professional School Counseling*, 12: 292–9.

Karcher, M J (2005)

The Effects of Developmental Mentoring and High School Mentors' Attendance on their Younger Mentees' Self-esteem, Social Skills, and Connectedness. *Psychology in the Schools*, 42: 65–77.

Klem, A M and Connell, J P (2004)

Relationships Matter: Linking Teacher Support to Student Engagement and Achievement. *Journal of School Health*, 74(7): 262–73.

141

Kokkinos, C M, Panayiotou, G and Davazoglou, A M (2005)
Correlates of Teacher Appraisals of Student Behaviors. *Psychology in the Schools*, 42(1): 79–89.

Lassander M, Hintsanen M, Suominen S, Mullola S, Vahlberg T and Volanen S M (2021)
Effects of School-Based Mindfulness Intervention on Health-Related Quality of Life: Moderating Effect of Gender, Grade, and Independent Practice in Cluster Randomized Controlled Trial. *Quality of Life Research*, 30(12): 3407–19.

Lewis S J, Arseneault L, Caspi A, Fisher H L, Matthews T, Moffitt T E, Odgers C L, Stahl D, Teng J Y and Danese A (2019)
The Epidemiology of Trauma and Post-Traumatic Stress Disorder in a Representative Cohort of Young People in England and Wales. *Lancet Psychiatry*, 6(3): 247–56.

Lilley, C, Ball, R and Vernon, H (2014)
The Experiences of 11–16 Year Olds on Social Networking Sites. London: NSPCC.

Lindsay, G and Dockrell, J (2012)
The Relationship Between Speech, Language and Communication Needs (SLCN) and Behavioural, Emotional and Social Difficulties. London: Department for Education.

Linsell, L, Johnson, S, Wolke, D, Morris, J, Kurinczuk, J J and Marlow, N (2019)
Trajectories of Behavior, Attention, Social and Emotional Problems from Childhood to Early Adulthood Following Extremely Preterm Birth: A Prospective Cohort Study. *European Child & Adolescent Psychiatry*, 28(4): 531–42.

Lloyd, M (2018)
Domestic Violence and Education: Examining the Impact of Domestic Violence on Young Children, Children, and Young People and the Potential Role of Schools. *Frontiers in Psychology*, 9. [online] Available at: www.frontiersin.org/articles/10.3389/fpsyg.2018.02094/full (accessed 2 April 2024).

Long, E (2022)
The Future of Pastoral Care in Schools: Exploring Whole-school Trauma-informed Approaches. *Pastoral Care in Education*, 40(3): 342–51.

Luthar S S (1993)
Annotation: Methodological and Conceptual Issues in the Study of Resilience. *Journal of Child Psychology and Psychiatry*, 34: 441–53.

Luthar, S S (2006)
Resilience in Development: A Synthesis of Research Across Five Decades, in Cicchetti, D and Cohen, D J (eds) *Development Psychopathology: Risk, Disorder and Adaptation* (pp 739–95). Hoboken, NJ: Wiley.

Maslow, A H (1943)
A Theory of Human Motivation. *Psychological Review*, 50(4): 370–96.

McCarthy, C J, Lambert, R G, Lineback, S, Fitchett, P and Baddouh, P G (2016)
Assessing Teacher Appraisals and Stress in the Classroom: Review of the Classroom Appraisal of Resources and Demands. *Educational Psychology Review*, 28(3): 577–603.

McMahon, E, Corcoran, P, O'Regan, G, Keeley, H, Cannon, M. et al (2017)
Physical Activity in European Adolescents and Associations with Anxiety, Depression and Well-being. *European Child & Adolescent Psychiatry*, 26(1): 111–22.

Madigan, D J and Kim, L E (2021)
Towards an Understanding of Teacher Attrition: A Meta-analysis of Burnout, Job Satisfaction, and Teachers' Intentions to Quit. *Teaching and Teacher Education,* 105: 1–14.

Maguire, M, Gewirtz, S, Towers, E and Neumann, E (2019)
Contextualising Policy Work: Policy Enactment and the Specificities of English Secondary Schools. *Research Papers in Education*, 35(4): 488–509.

Malecki, C K and Elliott, S N (2002)
Children's Social Behaviors as Predictors of Academic Achievement: A Longitudinal Analysis. *School Psychology Quarterly*, 17: 1–23.

Manning, A, Brock, R and Towers, E (2020)
Responding to Research: An Interview Study of the Teacher Well-being Support Being Offered in Ten English Schools. *Journal of Social Science Education*, 19(2): 75–94.

Manning, C and Gregoire, A (2009)
Effects of Parental Mental Illness on Children. *Psychiatry*, 8: 7–9.

Masten, A S (2001)
Ordinary Magic: Resilience Processes in Development. *American Psychologist*, 56(3): 227–38.

Masten, A and Garmezy, N (1985)

Risk, Vulnerability, and Protective Factors in Developmental Psychopathology, in Lahey, B B and Kazdin, A E (eds) *Advances in Clinical Child Psychology* (pp 1–52). New York: Plenum Press.

Maynard, B R, Farina, A, Dell, N A and Kelly, M S (2019)

Effects of Trauma-informed Approaches in Schools: A Systematic Review. *Campbell Systematic Review*, 15: 1–2.

Mental Health First Aid England (MHFA) (2018)

Adult Mental Health Aware Half Day Course Manual, MHFA England.

Mental Health First Aid (MHFA) (2020)

Mental Health Statistics. [online] Available at: https://mhfaengland.org/mhfa-centre/research-and-evaluation/mental-health-statistics/ (accessed 9 July 2024).

Mental Health Foundation (MHF) (2016)

Fundamental Facts about Mental Health 2016. London: Mental Health Foundation.

Mental Health Foundation (MHF) (2023)

Racism and Mental Health. London: Mental Health Foundation. [online] Available at: www.mentalhealth.org.uk/explore-mental-health/blogs/racism-and-mental-health (accessed 2 April 2024).

Mental Health Foundation (MHF) (2024)

The Mental Health of Asylum Seekers and Refugees in the UK. [online] Available at: www.mentalhealth.org.uk/sites/default/files/2024-02/MHF_Mental-Health-of-Asylum-Seekers_REPORT_A4_SINGLE-PAGES_0.pdf (accessed 31 July 2024).

Messiou, K and Azaola, M (2018)

A Peer-mentoring Scheme for Immigrant Students in English Secondary Schools: A Support Mechanism for Promoting Inclusion? *International Journal of Inclusive Education*, 22(2): 142–57.

Meyer, I H (2003)

Prejudice, Social Stress, and Mental Health in Lesbian, Gay and Bisexual Populations: Conceptual Issues and Research Evidence. *Psychological Bulletin*, 129: 674–97.

Mruk, C (1999)

Self-Esteem: Research, Theory and Practice. London: Free Association Books.

Mudaly, V and Sukhdeo, S (2015)

Mathematics Learning in the Midst of School Transition from Primary to Secondary School. *International Journal of Educational Sciences*, 11(3): 244–52.

Nathaniel, P, Sandilos, L E, Pendergast, L and Mankin, A (2016)

Teacher Stress, Teaching-Efficacy, and Job Satisfaction in Response to Test-based Educational Accountability Policies. *Learning and Individual Differences*, 50: 308–17.

National Education Union (NEU) (2019)

Supporting Trans and Gender Questioning Students. London: NEU. [online] Available at: https://neu.org.uk/advice/equality/lgbt-equality/supporting-trans-and-gender-questioning-students (accessed 2 April 2024).

National Education Union (NEU) (2021)

Turning the Page on Poverty: A Practical Guide for Education Staff to Help Tackle Poverty and the Cost of the School Day. [online] Available at: https://neu.org.uk/sites/default/files/2023-05/Turning%20the%20Page%20on%20Poverty.pdf (accessed 2 April 2024).

National Education Union (NEU) (2022)

Framework for Developing an Anti-Racist Approach. [online] Available at: https://neu.org.uk/latest/library/anti-racism-charter-framework-developing-anti-racist-approach (accessed 31 July 2024).

National Education Union (NEU) (2024)

Race Equality. [online] Available at: https://neu.org.uk/advice/equality/race-equality (accessed 23 April 2024).

National Health Service (NHS) (2005)

Mental Health of Children and Young People in Great Britain, 2004. [online] Available at: https://digital.nhs.uk/data-and-information/publications/statistical/mental-health-of-children-and-young-people-in-england/mental-health-of-children-and-young-people-in-great-britain-2004 (accessed 2 April 2024).

NHS Digital (2023)

Mental Health of Children and Young People in England, 2023: Wave 4 Follow Up to the 2017 Survey. [online] Available at: https://digital.nhs.uk/data-and-information/publications/statistical/mental-health-of-children-and-young-people-in-england/2023-wave-4-follow-up/part-1-mental-health (accessed 31 July 2024).

National Institute for Health and Care Excellence (NICE) (2013)

Social and Emotional Wellbeing for Children and Young People. London: NICE.

NSPCC (2015)

How Safe Are Our Children. [online] Available at: www.nspcc.org.uk/globalassets/documents/policy/england-briefing-priorities-how-safe-2015.pdf (accessed 2 April 2024).

Newlove-Delgado T, Marcheselli F, Williams T, Mandalia D, Dennes M, McManus S, Savic M, Treloar W, Croft K and Ford T (2023)
Mental Health of Children and Young People in England, 2023. Leeds: NHS England.

Nguyen, T D, Pham, L D, Crouch, M, and Springer, M G (2020)
The Correlates of Teacher Turnover: An Updated and Expanded Meta-Analysis of the Literature. *Educational Research Review*, 31: 100355.

Noble, C and Toft, M (2010)
Reducing Disaffection and Increasing School Engagement, in Aggleton, P, Dennison, C and Warwick, I (eds) *Promoting Health and Well-Being Through Schools* (pp 42–55). Abingdon: Routledge.

Office for National Statistics (ONS) (2015)
Measuring National Well-being: Insights into Children's Mental Health and Well-being. [online] Available at: www.ons.gov.uk/peoplepopulation andcommunity/wellbeing/articles/measuringnationalwellbeing/2015-10-20 (accessed 8 August 2018).

Office for National Statistics (ONS) (2016)
Internet Access – Households and Individuals: 2016. [online] Available at: www. ons.gov.uk/peoplepopulationandcommunity/householdcharacteristics/ homeinternetandsocialmediausage/bulletins/internetaccesshouseholdsand individuals/2016 (accessed 8 August 2018).

Office for Standards in Education (Ofsted) (2023)
The Annual Report of His Majesty's Chief Inspector of Education, Children's Services and Skills 2022/23. [online] Available at: www.gov.uk/ government/publications/ofsted-annual-report-202223-education- childrens-services-and-skills/the-annual-report-of-his-majestys-chief- inspector-of-education-childrens-services-and-skills-202223 (accessed 2 April 2024).

O'Hara, M (2014)
Teachers Left to Pick up Pieces from Cuts to Youth Mental Health Services. [online] Available at: www.theguardian.com/education/2014/ apr/15/pupils-mental-health-cuts-services-stress-teachers (accessed 8 August 2018).

Organisation for Economic Co-operation and Development (OECD) (2016)
PISA 2015 Results, Students' Wellbeing Volume III. OECD, April 2016. [online] Available at: www.oecd.org/edu/pisa-2015-results-volume-iii- 9789264273856-en.htm (accessed 15 July 2018).

Organisation for Economic Co-operation and Development, (OECD) (2020)

TALIS 2018 Results (Volume II) Teachers and School Leaders as Valued Professionals. [online] Available at: www.oecd.org/education/talis-2018-results-volume-ii-19cf08df-en.htm (accessed 2 February 2024).

Palmu, I R, Närhi, V M and Savolainen, H K (2018)

Externalizing Behaviour and Academic Performance – The Cross-lagged Relationship During School Transition. *Emotional and Behavioural Difficulties*, 23(2): 111–26.

Panayiotou, M, Ville, E, Poole, L, Gill, V and Humphrey, N (2020)

Learning from HeadStart: Does Cross-Age Peer Mentoring Help Young People with Emerging Mental Health Difficulties? London: EBPU.

Perfect, M M, Turley, M R, Carlson, J S, Yohanna, J and Saint Gilles, M P (2016)

School-related Outcomes of Traumatic Event Exposure and Traumatic Stress Symptoms in Students: A Systematic Review of Research from 1990 to 2015. *School Mental Health: A Multidisciplinary Research and Practice Journal*, 8(1): 7–43.

Perry, B D and Szalavitz, M (2006)

The Boy Who Was Raised as a Dog and Other Stories from a Child Psychiatrist's Notebook: What Traumatized Children Can Teach Us About Loss, Love, and Healing. New York: Basic Books.

Perry, B D and Winfrey, O (2021)

What Happened to You? Conversations on Trauma, Resilience, and Healing. London: Macmillan.

Peters, R and Brooks, R (2016)

Parental Perspectives on the Transition to Secondary School for Students with Asperger Syndrome and High Functioning Autism: A Pilot Survey Study. *British Journal of Special Education*, 43(1): 75–91.

Prever, M (2006)

Mental Health in Schools. London: Paul Chapman.

Public Health England (PHE) (2021)

Promoting Children and Young People's Mental Health and Well-being: A Whole School or College Approach. [online] Available at: https://assets.publishing.service.gov.uk/media/614cc965d3bf7f718518029c/Promoting_children_and_young_people_s_mental_health_and_well-being.pdf (accessed 2 April 2024).

Purtle, J (2020)

Systematic Review of Evaluations of Trauma-informed Organizational Interventions that include Staff Trainings. *Trauma, Violence, & Abuse*, 21(4): 725.

Raes, F, Griffith, J W, Van der Gucht, K and Williams, J M G (2014)
School-based Prevention and Reduction of Depression in Adolescents: A Cluster-randomized Controlled Trial of a Mindfulness Group Program. *Mindfulness*, 5(5): 477–86.

Reyes, A T, Andrusyszyn, M A, Iwaaiw, C, Forchuk, C and Babenko-Mould, Y (2015)
Resilience in Nursing Education: An Integrative Review. *Journal of Nursing Education*, 54(8): 438–44.

Ricarte, J J, Ros, L, Latorre, J M and Beltran, M T (2015)
Mindfulness-based Intervention in a Rural Primary School: Effects On Attention, Concentration and Mood. *International Journal of Cognitive Therapy*, 8(3): 258–70.

Roffey, S (2017)
Ordinary Magic Needs Ordinary Magicians: The Power and Practice of Positive Relationships for Building Youth Resilience and Wellbeing. *Kognition und Paedagogik*, 103: 38–57.

Rogers, C R (1951)
Client-centered Therapy. Boston: Houghton Mifflin.

Royal College of Paediatrics and Child Health (RCPCH) (2020)
State of Child Health. [online] Available at: https://stateofchildhealth.rcpch. ac.uk/evidence/mental-health/suicide/ (accessed 15 August 2024).

Royal Society for Public Health (RSPH) (2017)
#StatusOfMind: Social Media and Young People's Mental Health and Wellbeing. London: RSPH.

Ruggeri K, Garcia-Garzon E, Maguire Á, Matz S and Huppert F A (2020)
Well-being Is More Than Happiness and Life Satisfaction: A Multidimensional Analysis of 21 Countries. Health and Quality of Life Outcomes, 18(1): 192.

Sammons, P (2007)
A Review of School Effectiveness and Improvement. [online] Available at: www.cfbt.com/evidenceforeducation/pdf/Full%20Literature%20Review.pdf (accessed 8 August 2018).

Sanders, R (2020)

Care Experienced Children and Young People's Mental Health. [online] Available at: www.iriss.org.uk/resources/outlines/care-experienced-children-and-young-peoples-mental-health#:~:text=Care%20experienced%20children%20and%20young%20people%20have%20consistently,than%20one%20condition%20%28The%20Mental%20Health%20Foundation%2C%202002%29 (accessed 2 April 2024).

Sanderson, B and Brewer, M. (2017)

What Do We Know About Student Resilience in Health Professional Education? A Scoping Review of the Literature. *Nurse Education Today*, 58: 65–71.

Schonert-Reichl, K A and Lawlor, M S (2010)

The Effects of a Mindfulness-based Education Program on Pre- and Early Adolescents' Well-being and Social and Emotional Competence. *Mindfulness*, 1(3): 137–51.

Sciaraffa, M A, Zeanah, P D and Zeanah, C H (2017)

Understanding and Promoting Resilience in the Context of Adverse Childhood Experiences. *Early Childhood Education Journal*, 46(3): 343–53.

Serbin, L A, Stack, D M and Kingdon, D (2013)

Academic Success Across the Transition from Primary to Secondary Schooling Amongst Lower-Income Adolescents: Understanding the Effects of Family Resources and Gender. *Journal of Youth and Adolescence*, 42: 1331–47.

Sisask, M, Värnick, P, Värnik, A, Apter, A, Balazs, J, Balint, M and Wasserman, D (2014)

Teacher Satisfaction with School and Psychological Well-Being Affects Readiness to Help Children with Mental Health Problems. *Health Education Journal*, 73: 382–93.

Skaalvik, E and Skaalvik, S (2018)

Job Demands and Job Resources as Predictors of Teacher Motivation and Well-being. *Social Psychology of Education*, 21: 1251–75.

Sloan, S, Winter, K, Connolly, P and Gildea, A (2020)

The Effectiveness of Nurture Groups in Improving Outcomes for Young Children with Social, Emotional and Behavioural Difficulties in Primary Schools: An Evaluation of Nurture Group Provision in Northern Ireland. *Children and Youth Services Review*, 108 (104619): 1–11.

Sparling, E, Woods, K and Ford, A (2022)

Evaluation of an ACE-informed Whole-school Project Development. *Educational Psychology in Practice*, 38(1): 37–56.

Spenrath, M A, Clarke, M E and Kutcher, S (2011)

The Science of Brain and Biological Development: Implications for Mental Health Research, Practice and Policy. *Journal of the Canadian Academy of Child and Adolescent Psychiatry*, 20(4): 298–304.

Stapley, E, Town, R, Yoon, Y, Lereya, S T, Farr, J, Turner, J and Barnes, N (2022)

A Mixed Methods Evaluation of a Peer Mentoring Intervention in a UK school Setting: Perspectives from Mentees and Mentors. *Children and Youth Services Review*, 132, Article 106327.

Stephens, D (2013)

Teaching Professional Sexual Ethics Across the Seminary Curriculum. *Religious Education,* 108(2): 193–209.

Sterne, A and Poole, L (2010)

Domestic Violence and Children: A Handbook for Schools and Early Years Setting. London: Routledge.

Stewart-Brown, S (2006)

What is the Evidence on School Health Promotion in Improving Health or Preventing Disease and, Specifically, What is the Effectiveness of the Health Promoting Schools Approach? Copenhagen: WHO Regional Office for Europe.

Stonewall (2024)

List of LGBTQ+ Terms. [online] Available at: www.stonewall.org.uk/list-lgbtq-terms (accessed 23 April 2024).

Tait, M (2008)

Resilience as a Contributor to Novice Teacher Success, Commitment, and Retention. *Teacher Education Quarterly*, 35: 57–75.

Teo, A, Carlson, E, Mathieu, P J, Egeland, B and Sroufe, L A (1996)

A Prospective Longitudinal Study of Psychosocial Predictors of Academic Achievement. *Journal of School Psychology*, 34: 285–306.

Terjestam, Y, Bengtsson, H and Jansson, A (2016)

Cultivating Awareness at School. Effects on Effortful Control, Peer Relations and Well-being at School in Grades 5, 7, and 8. *School Psychology International*, 37(5): 456–69.

Thapa, A, Cohen, J Guffey, S and Alessandro, A (2013)

A Review of School Climate Research. *Review of Educational Research*, 83(3): 357–85.

Tiggemann, M and Slater A E (2014)
NetTweens: The Internet and Body Image Concerns in Preteenage Girls.
Journal of Early Adolescence, 34(5): 606–20.

Time to Change (2015)
Campaign Set to Tackle Life-Limiting Mental Health Stigma Among Teens.
[online] Available at: www.time-to-change.org.uk/news/new-campaign-
set-tackle-life-limiting-mental-health-stigma-among-teens (accessed 8
August 2018).

Towers, E, Gewirtz, S, Maguire, M and Neumann, E (2022)
A Profession in Crisis? Teachers' Responses to England's High-stakes
Accountability Reforms in Secondary Education. *Teaching and Teacher
Education*, 117.

**Tyler, R, Mannello, M, Mattingley, R, Roberts, C, Sage, R,
Taylor, S, Ward, M, Williams, S and Stratton, G (2016)**
Results from Wales' 2016 Report Card on Physical Activity for Children and
Youth: Is Wales Turning the Tide on Children's Inactivity? *Journal of Physical
Activity and Health*, 13(2 Suppl 2): S330–S336.

**Tymms, P B, Bolden, D S, Elliott, J G, Curtis, S E, Thomson, K
H, Dunn, C E et al (2016)**
Clustered Randomised Controlled Trial of Two Education Interventions
Designed to Increase Physical Activity and Well-being of Secondary School
Students: The MOVE Project. *BMJ Open*, 6(1): 1–11.

UNESCO Institute for Statistics (2016)
The World Needs Almost 69 Million New Teachers to Reach the
2030 Education Goals, No. 39 [online] Available at: http://uis.unesco.org/
sites/ default/files/documents/fs39-the-world-needs-almost-69-million-
new-teachers-to-reach-the-2030-education-goals-2016-en.pdf (accessed 13
August 2022).

Van der Kolk, B (2014)
*The Body Keeps the Score: Brain, Mind, and Body in the Healing
of Trauma*. New York: Viking.

**Vella, S A, Schranz, N K, Davernc, M, Hardy, L L, Hills,
A P, Morgan, P J, Plotnikoff, R C and Tomkinson, G (2016)**
The Contribution of Organised Sports to Physical Activity in Australia: Results
and Directions from the Active Healthy Kids Australia 2014 Report Card
on Physical Activity for Children and Young People. *Journal of Science and
Medicine in Sport*, 19: 407–12

Viglas, M and Perlman, M (2018)

Effects of a Mindfulness-based Program on Young Children's Self-regulation, Prosocial Behavior and Hyperactivity. *Journal of Child and Family Studies*, 27(4): 1150–61.

Vreeman R C and Carroll A E (2007)

A Systematic Review of School-Based Interventions to Prevent Bullying. *Archives of pediatrics & adolescent medicine*, 161(1): 78–88.

Weare, K (2010)

Promoting Mental Health Through Schools, in Aggleton, P, Dennison, C and Warwick, I (eds) *Promoting Health and Well-being Through Schools* (pp 24–41). Abingdon: Routledge.

Weare, K and Markham, W (2005)

What Do We Know About Promoting Mental Health Through Schools? *Promotion and Education*, 12: 118–22.

Welsh, M, Parke, R D, Widaman, K and O'Neil, R (2001)

Linkages Between Children's Social and Academic Competence: A Longitudinal Analysis. *Journal of School Psychology*, 39: 463–82.

Wentzel, K R (1993)

Does Being Good Make the Grade? Social Behavior and Academic Competence in Middle School. *Journal of Educational Psychology*, 85: 357–64.

West, P, Sweeting, H and Young, R (2010)

Transition Matters: Pupils' Experiences of the Primary–Secondary School Transition in the West of Scotland and Consequences for Well-Being and Attainment. *Research Papers in Education*, 25(1): 21–50.

West-Burnham, J (2009)

Developing outstanding leaders: Professional life Histories of outstanding headteachers: Full report 2009. London: National College for School Leadership.

Willis, P, Bland, R, Manka, L and Craft, C (2012)

The ABC of Peer Mentoring – What Secondary Students have to Say about Cross-age Peer Mentoring in a Regional Australian School. *Educational Research and Evaluation*, 18(2): 173–85.

Wood, J J (2006)

Effect of Anxiety Reduction on Children's School Performance and Adjustment. *Developmental Psychology*, 42: 345–9.

Woods, H C and Scott, H (2016)

#Sleepyteens: Social Media Use in Adolescence is Associated with Poor Sleep Quality, Anxiety, Depression and Low Self-esteem. *Journal of Adolescence*, 51: 41–9.

World Health Organisation (WHO) (2022)

Mental Health. [online] Available at: www.who.int/news-room/fact-sheets/detail/mental-health-strengthening-our-response (accessed 31 July 2024).

Yonezawa S, Jones M and Singer N R (2011)

Teacher Resilience in Urban Schools: The Importance of Technical Knowledge, Professional Community, and Leadership Opportunities. *Urban Education*, 46: 913–31.

Young Minds (2021)

The Impact of Covid-19 on Young People with Mental Health Needs. [online] Available at: www.youngminds.org.uk/about-us/reports-and-impact/coronavirus-impact-on-young-people-with-mental-health-needs/ (accessed 9 July 2024).

Young Minds (2024)

Mental Health Statistics. [online] Available at: www.youngminds.org.uk/about-us/media-centre/mental-health-statistics/#:~:text=One%20in%20six%20children%20aged,in%20every%20classroom%20(i). (accessed 31 July 2024).

Zins, J E, Bloodworth, M R, Weissberg, R P and Walberg, H J (2004)

The Scientific Base Linking Social and Emotional Learning to School Success, in Zins, J, Weissberg, R, Wang, M and Walberg, H J (eds) *Building Academic Success on Social and Emotional Learning: What Does the Research Say?* (pp 3–22). New York: Teachers College Press.

✛ INDEX